Alzheimer's

A Love Story

Alzheimer's

A Love Story

One Year in
My Husband's
Journey

Ann Davidson

A Birch Lane Press Book
Published by Carol Publishing Group

A Birch Lane Press Book
Published by Carol Publishing Group
Birch Lane Press is a registered trademark of Carol Communications, Inc.

Editorial, sales and distribution, rights and permissions inquiries should be addressed to Carol Publishing Group, 120 Enterprise Avenue, Secaucus, N.J. 07094

In Canada: Canadian Manda Group, One Atlantic Avenue, Suite 105, Toronto, Ontario M6K 3E7

Carol Publishing Group books may be purchased in bulk at special discounts for sales promotion, fund-raising, or educational purposes. Special editions can be created to specifications. For details, contact Special Sales Department, Carol Publishing Group, 120 Enterprise Avenue, Secaucus, N.J. 07094.

Manufactured in the United States of America
10 9 8 7 6 5 4 3 2 1

LIBRARY OF CONGRESS CATALOGING-IN-PUBLICATION DATA
Davidson, Ann, 1938–
    Alzheimer's, a love story: one year in my husband's journey / by Ann Davidson.
        p. cm.
    "A Birch Lane Press book."
    ISBN 1-55972-418-8 (HC)
    1. Davidson, Julian M.—Health.   2. Alzheimer's disease—Patients—Biography.   3. Davidson, Ann, 1938–   . I. Title.
RC523.2.D384D39   1997
362.1'96831'0092—dc21
[B]   96-51668
                                                                                CIP

For Julian

Contents ~

Contents

Contents

Acknowledgments ⁓

I am deeply grateful to many people for their help and encouragement in creating this book—and for the outpouring of support and affection given Julian and me.

Heartfelt thanks to the Monday Writers: Connie Crawford, Helen Bigelow, Maureen Eppstein, Henri Bensussen, Margaret Mullen, Sandy Raney, Louisa Rogers, and Amanda Kovattana, who listened to my stories, gave suggestions, and urged me on. Special thanks to Mary Jane Moffat and Dorothy Wall, inspiring and encouraging writing mentors; to Joan Bisagno, who gave me a quiet place; and to Bernie Roth, who handled my computer messes.

To Charles Familant for his generous, enduring support; to Helen Davies, Helen de Vries, and John Preston, for their compassion and counsel; to Carol Denehy and the dedicated staff at Rosener House, Julian's day care center; and to Beth Logan, of the Family Caregivers Alliance, I am forever grateful. I extend enormous respect to Verna Aldous and all the caregivers I've met who taught me about resilience.

I am especially grateful to Roseanne Strucinski, Bud Squier, Ray Clayton, Penny Bauer, Presocia Mirkil, Tom Forrest, and Paul Feder, who gave Julian gifts of music, walks, lunches, bike rides, and chocolate, and me the gift of time.

Among many caring friends, I want to thank Magda Gerber, Judy Squier, Ginny du Prau, Jan Feldman, Eileen Bobrow, Bernie and Ruth Roth, Irv and Ellen Zucker, Joan and Wise Allen, Anne Prescott and Joyce Fulton, Bence Gerber, Sita de Leeuw, Annaliese Korner, Rachelle Marshall, Hannah Berman, and Betty Brown, dear friends on this long journey.

Acknowledgments

I want to express my appreciation to Erla Smith, Julian's research associate, for her hard work and tireless loyalty, and Julian's staff at Stanford, who helped him conclude his professional life in a responsible way. Special thanks to Ben Sachs, Ray Rosen, Manuel Mas, John Bancroft, Jack Clarke, Marcia Stefanick, and Danusia Szumowski, among others, Julian's colleagues and friends.

Thanks to my sister Jean Colvin and brother-in-law Bharat Rawal, for their steadfast caring for our father, and to my cousins Dorothy Nasatir and Gene Piercy, for their many visits and calls.

Finally, deep appreciation, beyond words, to my very special family: our daughter, Karen de Sa, and her husband, Ronaldo (Beiçola) de Sa, our son Ben Davidson and our son-in-law Greg Riley, and our son Jeff Davidson, all of whom cheer me on and bring energy, love, and vitality into my life. And to my grandchildren, Antar, Celina, and Rasa de Sa, who already know much about Alzheimer's and the value of joy and play.

I want to also thank David Spiegel, M.D., for his special insights and for endorsing this work. Thank you to my editor, Hillel Black, who saw the promise and made this book happen.

Author to Reader ⁓

One day in August, 1990, I picked my husband up at the clinic after a spinal tap, part of a neurological exam for some vague, subtle memory problems Julian had been having. I didn't even have an appointment. I had been told only that Julian shouldn't ride his bike home after the procedure.

The test results wouldn't be available for a week. So when the doctor met me at the neurology desk and said, "Come in, I want to tell you something," I thought she'd give me instructions on what Julian should or shouldn't do after the spinal tap.

We walked into a little side room behind the nurses' station and stood facing each other. Immediately the doctor said, "Your husband has a primary progressive dementia. He won't have a normal life span. Dismantle his professional life as quickly as possible. Go out and get help for yourself. Decide if you want to tell him or not. He has a progressive brain disease, probably Alzheimer's."

I felt as if a train had hit me. A minute later, I was back in the hall and Julian emerged from the treatment room. I could barely look at him. I didn't know what to do or say. At that moment, I began keeping a terrible secret, something I'd never done in our thirty-year marriage.

Julian was fifty-nine, a physiology professor at Stanford University. I was fifty-two, a speech therapist, just recovered two years earlier from a mastectomy and six months of chemotherapy. Our three children, in their twenties, were out on their own. Until the doctor's words, Julian and I had been elated over our good fortune and the gift of freedom and health.

The doctor told me to telephone before Julian's next appointment and instruct her whether or not to tell him his diagnosis. After private, agonizing vacillation, I decided Julian wasn't ready to hear the words "Alzheimer's" or "dementia," at least not yet. Instead, when we met to officially get the test results, the doctor told Julian he had "neurologically based memory problems." She said the cause was unknown (a partial truth), and advised him to eliminate stress and ease out of his demanding work. She cautiously answered what few questions Julian asked.

After that meeting, Julian and I talked endlessly about what to do. With great disappointment, Julian canceled a long-planned lecture tour to Israel, realizing that ten lectures would be impossible. I urged him to let his associate teach his upcoming classes and his postdoctoral fellow present already scheduled papers. I struggled with whether or not to tell his colleagues the diagnosis behind his back.

Still keeping the terrible secret, I awakened at night with panic attacks. I became so anxious that I asked my oncologist for the first tranquilizers of my life. I sought out a psychiatrist specializing in self-hypnosis to learn a tool to help me calm down.

Of course, I told our three children. In awkward phone calls, I described the findings of "neurological memory problems," once again afraid to say "Alzheimer's." To protect them from my own overwhelming fear, I told them that nothing would change suddenly and that we had time.

Gradually I revealed more, until eventually I told them the actual diagnosis. Our daughter and sons were stunned. I wrote Julian's family in Scotland and Israel and gradually told a few close friends. Each time I said the word "Alzheimer's," I felt as if I were establishing the fact.

Those first weeks after Julian's diagnosis, I watched him read physiology journals on the sofa and imagined him slumped in a wheelchair, drooling. I pictured him wandering the neighborhood at night in pajamas, being brought home by the police. I imagined him sitting on the floor playing with blocks, as a cousin's father with Alzheimer's had done. Or deteriorating quickly in a year and dying in a nursing home as this same cousin's husband had done.

I imagined Julian making love to me and afterward asking, "Who are you?" I couldn't imagine life without him.

For months I grieved and mourned, even though Julian was right there, strong and alive, warm and breathing, wrapped around me in bed each night. Petty grudges melted away, and I appreciated him as in our early days together, loving him with a fierce passion I hadn't felt in years. I was tormented with the questions of when and how to tell him his fate.

Then, one day, Julian received a letter asking him to come to the Department of Motor Vehicles. No reason was stated. When he stood at the counter and asked why he'd been summoned, the clerk said simply, "You have Alzheimer's."

"Alzheimer's?" Julian shouted at the bewildered clerk. "I'm a professor at Stanford! My secretary is in the car! What do you mean, Alzheimer's?"

Julian came home white-faced, shattered, and told me what happened. We sat on the couch with the truth before us.

"I know, darling, I know," I whispered. "But I couldn't tell you before." He stared at me and slowly nodded. We fell against each other and lay in each other's arms, not knowing what to say.

Later I learned that California law requires doctors to report all Alzheimer's diagnoses to the Department of Motor Vehicles, which routinely summons patients for a driving assessment. They permitted Julian to drive for another year. But I knew none of this at the time.

After that, Julian's problems became the topic of nearly all conversation. We talked endlessly about how he should disengage from Stanford in a responsible way. He knew he needed to make changes, but he wasn't ready to tell others why.

"People will think I'm a freak," Julian said. "Alzheimer's has a terrible stigma. It's not like other diseases."

As his staff began taking a larger role in running his research, Julian vacillated between relief that he no longer had to perform at a level that was now too difficult and deep sadness over leaving his career. Fear hung over him: Who would he be now?

Already Alzheimer's was eroding our lives by stealing Julian's language and intellect—much of what had attracted me to him. He forgot names, spoke in vague, rambling circumlocutions, and repeated himself. Who would Julian be, stripped of his precise and articulate speech? We were wordy people: reading, discussing, writing, analyzing, comparing, arguing, sharing. We didn't go fishing, work in gardens, build bookcases, play cards, or make music. We talked.

Although Julian said "salt" for "pepper," "library" for "bookstore," and "he" for "she," in many ways he continued to be an active, functioning man. But I never knew what he understood or remembered, what he could or couldn't do. He handled his fears by putting his decline way off in the future. "So what if I'm in a nursing home when I'm eighty?" he said.

Chaos crept into our lives: lost keys, missed appointments, unpaid bills, misplaced glasses. I felt Julian sliding into a black abyss, and I was sliding with him. The dark thought pulsed through my head: "We're going down."

Searching for information and guidance, I was terrified by what I read in Alzheimer's pamphlets:

> Alzheimer's Disease is a progressive, degenerative disease that attacks the brain and results in impaired memory, thinking and behavior. . . . Problems remembering recent events and difficulty performing familiar tasks are early symptoms. . . . The Alzheimer's patient may experience confusion, personality change, behavior change, impaired judgment, and difficulty finding words, finishing thoughts, or following directions. . . . The disease eventually leaves its victims totally unable to care for themselves.

". . . totally unable to care for themselves." I couldn't get those words out of my mind.

The material I read seemed aimed at families whose loved ones were in more advanced stages than Julian. Books entitled *The Thirty-Six-Hour Day*, *The Loss of Self*, and *The Long Bereavement* sat on the library shelf. I couldn't even open them. There seemed little available for people like us, newly diagnosed with Alzheimer's. Many books stated that the caregiver is the second victim, whose life is also destroyed.

But it's a long way from diagnosis to oblivion. How did people get through those years? How did they manage? I began seeking advice from groups and agencies.

One day I sat on the psychiatrist's couch, deep in a hypnosis session, my chest tight, my heart pounding, my breath in short gasps. "Tell me what you see," this wise man said. And I described the fierce images: Julian drooling, babbling, incontinent, wandering, mute, lying for years in a fetal position. I saw myself helpless and alone. My chest heaved in great sobs. "He's going down," I cried. "Both of us are going down."

"Breathe," the psychiatrist said. "Breathe deeply. Now tell me what you want."

And in a flash I saw clearly that what I wanted was to "go down" in a spirit of love—not fear and anger, no matter what transpired.

Brave words for someone barely started on this terrible journey. But that day something shifted. Clinging to that hope, I began to write. I told Julian I was writing about how Alzheimer's affected us. "Even that I sometimes yell at you," I said. "Do it," he said, giving me his blessing.

When I began writing, Julian was in the "mild-moderate" stage; I was still a stumbling beginner in dealing with Alzheimer's. Yet I needed to record what I was learning about commitment, loss, acceptance, and love. I needed to make sense of our precarious days.

I wrote while waiting for Julian outside his speech therapy sessions, his counseling appointments, the dentist's office. I wrote in stolen half hours in restaurants and cafes; while he watched television or took a nap. In spite of the short, fragmented writing periods, I filled page after page. Over the next twelve months, this book emerged.

So here is our tale—one year in our lives with Alzheimer's. A frightening year, a heartbreaking year, and a year of growth, with acceptance, moments of humor and joy, and an odd sort of peace. . . . *Alzheimer's, A Love Story.*

Summer 1992

That's what we were doing now . . .
preparing for his silence.

A Quiet Buddha

We drove into Kit Carson Lodge just after sunset. "Our cabin faces Silver Lake," I told our son Ben. "From your bed you can watch the dawn pinken Thunder Mountain." Ben was home from graduate school to spend the summer with Julian and me, and we brought him for a week to our favorite mountains.

I parked the car by the path to the cabin. Thick Jeffrey pines lined the path, their branches nodding in the evening breeze. The gray-green lake rippled with wavy lines. Julian, Ben, and I unloaded the duffel bags and grocery boxes. We placed our fruit in the basket, laid our green checkered cloth on the round wooden table, set our books on the bookcase, hung our towels on the hooks, put our food on the shelf, claiming this rented cabin as our own. "Mackinaw" was ours for a week.

"We'll have quiet times every morning," we told each other. "We'll read and write. Then we'll hike in the afternoons. We'll go to Lake Winnemucca, take the trail from Carson Pass. We'll climb Elephant's Back, cross-country. Maybe go up Round Top Peak." Julian and I have come for years to Silver Lake, high in the Sierra south of Lake Tahoe. Excitedly we planned sharing these loved places with Ben.

I described the terrain while we made dinner. Broiled fresh lingcod. Sweet white corn bought that afternoon at a vegetable stand in the Central Valley. Juicy tomatoes with chopped green onions. Blackberries with vanilla yoghurt.

As it was Friday night, I lit two candles and chanted the traditional Hebrew blessing. I covered my eyes with my hands like an Orthodox Jewish woman, which I rarely do. "*Baruch Atah Adonai* . . .," I said, "*melech ha'olam.* . . ."

If I really think about these words, I don't believe them. "Praised are You, Lord our God, King of the universe. . . ." The words in Jewish prayers often put up barriers for me. But I do believe in pausing a moment over our food and over this gathering. Here in this cabin with a whole week in the mountains before us, Julian, Ben, and me together, healthy and present in this timeless moment. Reciting ancient Hebrew words feels good if I don't think about their translation.

Julian mumbled the blessing over wine and bread, stumbling over words he once knew so well. To our surprise, Ben finished the kiddush. He sang the full blessing. We didn't even realize he remembered it. Then we ate our cod, corn, and tomatoes and reminisced over other Friday nights when the kids were young.

"I remember so many Fridays," Ben said, "when you, Mom, lit candles and made a good dinner and we'd eat in the dining room. Dad said kiddush. And you'd insist that we eat with you even if we had plans for later."

He said this with some fondness. I felt relieved, remembering the hassles to get the kids to eat with us on Friday nights when they were pushing to go out on their own. I remembered how tired I had felt, all the rushing and scrambling and arguing in those years.

Over dinner, we talked about Judaism in Julian's childhood in Scotland, why he stopped being religious, how he lived in relation to his Orthodox background, and what he had wanted for his children in California.

Julian's speech faltered. He didn't always use the right word, and he often paused in the middle of a phrase. I helped him out at times, filling in words, finishing his fragmented sentences. But the discussion flowed.

A good dinner conversation, I thought. We talked easily, no stress, no tension. In spite of his hesitations and word-finding problems, Julian fully participated, or so I believed.

But as we lingered over coffee, Julian suddenly left the table and lay down on the couch. He said he didn't feel well. He went into the bedroom, put on his pajamas, and got into bed.

I went in to him. He was sitting in bed with the blanket pulled up over his face. "Are you sick?" I said. "What is it?"

He pulled the covers higher over his head.

"Leave me alone," he mumbled.

"Julian, have I hurt your feelings? Have I offended you? Did I say something to hurt you?" Maybe Julian felt upset by Ben criticizing the government policies in Israel during the Intifada.

No comment.

"Tell me," I urged. "Tell me what's wrong." I shut the pine door of the bedroom. In the kitchen I heard Ben rattling pots, washing the dishes.

"I'm no good." Julian's muffled voice came from under the blanket. "I'm just no good anymore. I can't do anything."

I wrapped my arms around the blankety lump. I pulled the covers away from his face and ruffled his hair. "I admire you so much," I said. "I respect you. Remember that." It's shitty to live with memory problems, I told him. Accepting any disease is hard, but especially Alzheimer's. "It's not your fault.

"Of course you feel depressed sometimes. You have every right to feel sad. But this feeling will pass. We'll have many good times, too." I hugged him tight. "I love you," I said. "Ben loves you. Remember that."

I went out to the cabin's main room and put in a cassette—a tape of Sephardic songs that Ben had recorded for Julian as a gift. The sweet, melancholy voice of Victoria de los Angeles drifted into the bedroom.

"There's beautiful music to listen to," I said. Julian lay in bed motionless. The blanket was off his head, now tucked under his chin, but his face looked sad in the dim light.

I stepped outside to check if the music was too loud for the adjacent cabin. The black canopy overhead was sprinkled with bright stars, and dark pines pointed toward the tiny lights dotting the sky.

Ben joined me on the deck. "Is Dad okay?" he asked softly. I told him what Julian had said about being no good. Ben fell silent. In the darkness I saw him wipe his hand across his eye.

"Maybe it's because we were laughing in the car," Ben said. "Dad probably thought we were laughing at him. Humor relieves the tension, but we shouldn't laugh at him."

I knew exactly what Ben was thinking about. While driving through the foothills, Julian told us he had talked that morning with Erla, the research associate in his lab at Stanford. They had been discussing our trip. Julian said he was surprised that Erla had never heard of Lake Tahoe and didn't know where it was. Only he wasn't saying "Tahoe." He called it "Tee-ha" or "To-hee" or "Tee-ta." Picturing the scene, I had laughed. I imagined Julian telling Erla we were going to Lake Tee-ha and Erla telling him she had never heard of Lake Tee-ha and asking where it was. I wasn't laughing at Julian, it was the situation.

"I didn't mean to hurt him," I told Ben. "It just seemed so funny."

"Let's be sensitive this week," he said.

"Yes, and let's be careful not to exclude him."

"It's hard, Mom," Ben confessed. "I get tired listening to him. Sometimes I just space out and don't pay attention."

"I know," I said. "It's hard to talk with him for long periods of time. Can you imagine how I feel alone with him for days on end? But he's very sensitive to people pulling away and not wanting to be with him."

Back in the cabin, I helped Ben make his bed. Then I went into our room and shut the door. I put on my nightgown and slipped into bed beside Julian. I unbuttoned his top pajama button and lay my cheek against the curly hairs on his chest, pressing my body hard against his. He felt warm and familiar. The voice of Victoria de los Angeles drifted in, haunting and sad. Little bells tinkled in the background against the strums of a guitar.

"There are many quiet people in the world," I whispered. "It's not bad to be a quiet person—only you haven't been one before. You're used to being a lively, quick, center-of-the-conversation person. Being quiet is new for you," I said. "Let's find good images of quiet people."

"I love you." Julian stroked my hair. "I know I'll always have you. But what can I do? Who will I be?"

Tears rolled down my cheeks. We lay under the clean white sheets, holding each other, listening to the singer's melancholy voice. I named our quiet friends. Suddenly I remembered the small gray soapstone carving of a Buddha which sits on Julian's cluttered desk above piles of papers, in front of his dictionaries and thesaurus, in front of all the lost words. The Buddha sits cross-legged above the chaos of papers on Julian's desk, a serene expression on his face, hands folded in his lap.

"You could just sit quietly," I said, "and learn to be a smiling Buddha."

Father and Son

Looking through binoculars, I watch their two figures move slowly up the steep trail. In my circles of vision, I see Ben climbing ahead, a white shirt tied around his waist, his blue shorts moving higher and higher up the switchbacks. Julian climbs several yards behind him, wearing khaki pants and a green shirt. They have almost reached the snow patch. Beyond the snow loom the jagged volcanic rocks of Round Top Peak.

Ben and Julian are climbing Round Top today, the highest peak in this wilderness area, the one Fremont climbed in the days of Kit Carson. From it you can see north over Meiss Meadow to Lake Tahoe. You can see south over layers of Sierra ridges and valleys. Looking east, you see the lower ranges east of Carson Pass; you see the huge gray sloping bare hump of Elephant's Back. Looking west, the large blue patch of Caples Lake and Silver Lake below that. Round Top is a power place.

Today, I'm hanging out at a small icy circle of dark water at the foot of craggy cliffs of volcanic rock, surrounded by large patches of sparkling white snow. Water tumbles into Round Top Lake from the melting snow patch above. Tall grass borders the north shore where I wait, sprawled at times on some granite outcropping near the lake, or, when the mosquitos buzz around me too much, on short tough meadow grass farther away from the water.

Through the round lenses, I watch Julian limp up the switchbacks several yards behind Ben. I see his uneven gait as he picks his way slowly around boulders, the space between Ben and Julian widening. Watching them climb, I see the strength of my handsome son. I see his aging father limping behind. They are climbing this peak together.

Summer 1992

I didn't go because I wanted Julian and Ben to have this adventure, father and son, without me.

They have worked their way up the switchbacks and are skirting the edge of the larger snow patch. Now Julian and Ben are silhouetted on the ridge, two black sticks against the sky.

Ben begins climbing the dark volcanic rocks that form Round Top while Julian stands alone, a small, dark figure against endless blue. Ben scrambles over large boulders, his white shirt flapping around his waist. Julian remains standing on the ridge. It looks as though he's not going all the way to the top.

Three years ago, Julian climbed Round Top by himself; now, less than two years after his diagnosis, I'm afraid for him to hike alone. He might get lost, lose the trail, or make a poor judgement about what's safe. His capable son is leading the way. The difference between their pace and postures astonishes me.

Ben is patient with Julian these days. He defers to him when Julian wants to speak, asking, "What did you say, Dad?" if two of us talk at once. He acknowledges Julian's remarks. "That's interesting, Dad," or "I didn't know that." He speaks in a voice full of respect and compassion. He's considerate of Julian's needs, sensitive to where he is and whether he needs help.

Gone are the snappy, irritable, competitive tones of Ben's adolescence. Gone is the strident, urgent quality that so characterized Ben's and Julian's conversations for years, all those political arguments about Nicaragua, El Salvador, Cuba, and the Soviet Union, Ben's Marxist views more intense than Julian's. Liberal Julian somehow turned into a conservative enemy.

For years they jockeyed and struggled against each other, each stubborn, each needing to be right and to prove the other wrong. They locked horns, like two bull elk, and the house rocked with their arguments, about politics, the economy, the FBI and the CIA.

Now Ben is gentle with Julian and understanding with me.

When he tells us about graduate school, the papers he's writing and seminars he's giving, I know he misses talking to the bright, articulate man his father used to be. I know he yearns for a sensible, poignant, relevant conversation, instead of the vague, superficial remarks they currently exchange.

"It's so different now, Mom," Ben told me when we were alone. "Living with Dad this past month, I see the changes so clearly. I couldn't really see it before."

Our talks are bland, rambling, and simple. We all miss the interesting tangles we used to have, the intricate verbal snarls we'd work our way out of. Ben has grown up and become his own person, no longer needing to assert himself constantly against his father. How I wish they could now really talk.

Ben has disappeared into the huge black boulders which form Round Top. Through the binoculars, I watch Julian sitting on the ridge, his back toward me, looking out over the southern view. Finally Ben reappears, slowly picking his way down from the summit. He joins Julian and the two are poised for a moment on the ridge, two dark lines against the sky.

Then they descend the steep trail, around the snow patch and down the switchbacks. Their figures grow larger and larger in the binocular lens: their bare chests, their shirts tied around their waists, their jerky gait as they lurch down the trail, growing to human scale as they descend.

I hear their boots crunching on gravel, hear them talking and laughing there on the other side of the willows. They're back, faces red and sweaty, chests glistening. They tell me what they have seen from the ridge. I unscrew the top from the plastic bottle and offer them water.

The three of us head down the winding, flower-decked trail toward our car, parked at Woods Lake, and then drive toward Silver Lake, toward home.

"What's Hope and What's Denial?"

Waves from Silver Lake slapped up on the sandy beach below our cabin. Wind shooshed through the pines. A squirrel screeched and two jays flew after each other around the thick trunk of the fir just beyond the deck rails. The wind cooled my face as I tried to quiet myself alone on the deck.

Julian, Ben, and I just had our first tense time. I don't even know what caused it. I was doing the overdue bills, with my usual annoyance. Part of me still wishes Julian could handle the finances, as he did for thirty years. One thought led to another and I started fretting about our long-term financial problems in a vague, wordless way.

When I pointed out Ben's long-distance calls on the phone bill, he snapped, "Okay. I'll pay you for them. Shall I write you a check right now?" Both of us knew that it was reasonable for him to pay for his long-distance calls, but old buttons were pushed.

Julian had been irritable ever since I'd read him parts of the book *My Journey Into Alzheimer's*, a young minister's personal story of early-stage dementia. Over breakfast I'd read carefully selected sections in which the author describes what Julian experiences too, thoughts flying away, words disappearing, confusion in crowds, trouble reading and calculating, embarrassment, and fear of failing. I thought it might help Julian to hear someone else's struggle. But he became dejected and long-faced, not finding it helpful at all.

As I was finishing the bills Julian's questions started over and over: where was his wallet, his shoe, his pills, the milk. I answered sharply; Ben responded impatiently too. Julian stomped out and walked to the little store a few hundred yards from our cabin. While he was gone and while Ben took a shower, I tried to calm down by sitting alone outside for a few minutes instead of tidying the cabin.

Julian returned from the store, climbed the steps, and asked again what he was supposed to buy. He had forgotten he was going for bread. When he returned a second time, he slammed down the loaf and stomped out again, his face long and sad. His head hung down and he limped along the road by the lake. Ben leapt down the steps and caught up with him, and I watched the two blue-jeaned figures walking side by side, glad to see Ben sensitive and responsive to Julian's mood.

Soon Ben came back to the cabin alone and Julian continued limping toward the lake, his head jutting forward, his whole body drooped.

"He's upset, isn't he?" I said the obvious to Ben, who dropped down beside me on the blue plastic chair.

"He says you read some terrible things. Dad said, 'Everything's different now.' He says he didn't know it was that bad. He'll have to 'think it through.'"

"But I didn't read him anything he doesn't already know," I protested. "I didn't read the depressing parts."

I didn't read the descriptions of the author's fears of having his brain turn to mush, or his despair over his IQ, which had fallen to half what it was, or how he feared giving up independence and needing to be cared for. I had read these parts earlier myself, stony faced and shivering, yet morbidly curious about these awesome possibilities.

I didn't read Julian what the author wrote of his terror over descending into blackness, living in a smaller and smaller "playpen of safety," becoming a babbling, or mute, nonknowing shell of a man, a man whose body is there but whose spirit, whose soul, whose self has slowly slipped away and gone. I didn't read him those sections.

"I only read what Dad experiences too," I defended myself to Ben. "I thought it would help him feel better to know how others with memory problems cope."

Ben leaned back in the deck chair, stretched out his legs, and propped his feet on the rail, interlacing his fingers behind his curly brown hair, still damp from the shower.

"The author of that book is young, like Dad, in his fifties, the minister of a large congregation," I continued. "He's also struggling to develop a positive attitude and find ways to live with Alzheimer's as best he can."

"But Dad doesn't want to think about Alzheimer's," Ben said. "He knows, but he has a lot of denial going. He copes by denying."

"Yes, he does," I said. "He feels better by telling himself, 'Oh, maybe I'll be in a nursing home when I'm eighty.' Or, 'Who knows what will happen to any of us.' Or, 'Maybe everyone doesn't become mute.' Why shouldn't he tell himself that?"

"Dad doesn't realize how handicapped he really is," Ben added.

"Maybe that's a blessing," I said. "Denial wards off unbearable anxiety. Why shouldn't he be as hopeful as he can?" I looked into Ben's clear blue eyes, so like Julian's, and at his angular, tanned face.

"What's hope and what's denial?" I asked Ben, gazing out at the lake's gray water. "What's the healthiest mixture? Dad's 'denial' isn't hurting anyone. It isn't preventing us from doing what we need to do." I told Ben we'd been to an attorney and prepared a trust, a will, powers of attorney for health care and for legal and financial matters. Julian was extricating himself from his duties at Stanford in a responsible and dignified way. He was driving less and now let me drive without making a fuss. As long as he acknowledged what was going on and behaved safely, then what was the problem with denial, if it helped him cope?

Ben stared out at Silver Lake, then looked at me with soft eyes. An enormous sense of gratitude welled up: I have this kind and gentle son to talk to.

Then we went into the cabin and began making lunch. Ben made tuna sandwiches while I put oranges into our packs and filled the plastic water bottles. Julian clumped up the stairs and entered the cabin. No one referred to what had happened; we just got busy preparing our hike.

The usual discussion over what to wear: long pants or shorts? Should we take a jacket or poncho? Do we think it might rain? Is a sweater too heavy? Shall I carry the camera, the binoculars, or both? Should I take my journal in case they climb a mountain and I sit by a lake?

We finally got the gear together, zipped our packs, and left for the hike from Woods Lake to Winnemucca, then up the barren, rocky pass to Round Top Basin. We planned today to go over the ridge to the lake on the other side. Before leaving, we iced Julian's toes and he took an anti-inflammatory pill to ease the arthritis in his feet. The pill seemed to work: He walked without limping.

The sky was overcast and a chilling wind blew as we started up the trail. Mule ears in meadows presented yellow flowers that hadn't been there two days before. Things change fast in the

Sierra. Yellow blossoms covered the hillsides, and tiny white flowers, like little stars, clung to granite. Wandering daisies grew along rushing streams.

We climbed higher, puffing less than earlier in the week when we'd hiked this trail. We looked back across the open valley to Red Lake Peak and ahead at snow patches on Round Top's jagged cliffs, which two days ago Ben and Julian had climbed.

As we left Winnemucca and started up the pass toward Round Top Lake, the sky suddenly darkened to a steel gray. Above the timberline, we hiked over smooth slabs of granite strewn with boulders. The wind grew colder and drops of rain plopped on our heads. Suddenly thunder boomed, echoing in the rocky basin. White lightning bolts streaked down the dark sky toward Elephant's Back, not far away. We stared at the lightning as rain drops turned to hail, pelting our faces. We tore into our packs, pulling out ponchos. Should we stand near the solitary wind-twisted pines that dotted the basin? we asked each other. Or crouch by a boulder? Lightning streaks lit up the sky fearfully close.

Our blue ponchos draped over us, we huddled near a granite boulder. "Let's get out of here," I yelled, as another lightning bolt crashed over Elephant's Back.

Julian, Ben and I turned and ran back toward Woods Lake, their two lumpy blue shapes bouncing ahead of me down the trail. We shrieked at each clap of thunder, yelled with each bolt of lightning. We didn't really know how to protect ourselves, except to leave this exposed place.

Scampering down the trail, we considered death by lightning: Would it hurt? Would you feel burned? Would it happen fast? We ran and howled and laughed and shrieked as thunder clapped and pellets of ice stung our faces. Only when the trail dropped into the shelter of a fir forest did I stop being anxious.

The wind quieted and the hail stopped. My heart rate returned to normal and my breathing eased. We strode leisurely down the trail, passing ice pellets piled in crannies by granite boulders and beside marsh marigolds growing in black mud near the streams.

Quick, cold, sharp, stinging—the storm had passed. Washed clean, pines and firs and mule ears glistened green in the new bright sun. Julian's face looked calm and relaxed. Ben made wisecracks and he and Julian joked and horsed around. We threw our wet ponchos in the back of the station wagon and drove down Highway 88 to the worn, wooden Kirkwood Inn, where we sat in captain's chairs around a red-and-white-checkered table and ordered hot blueberry pie and coffee. The storm was over.

The Death of Little Kenny Miller

The small headline in the lower right corner of yesterday's *San Francisco Chronicle* leapt out: "Boy Found Dead in High Sierra."

Kenny Miller, age twelve, was found dead by hikers high on a ridge near Steven's Peak overlooking Meiss Meadow near Carson Pass. He'd been missing for eleven days after wandering away from his parents and sister on a day's outing to the meadow, the article said. A full-scale search had continued for a week and had been called off only three days ago.

Julian, Ben, and I had seen that search: the rescue teams, dogs, and helicopters. On Wednesday, in the middle of our week at Silver Lake, we had decided to hike up the ridge from Schneider Cow Camp. The wildflowers were like a garden, the trail guide said, and you could see magnificent views from the pass.

Driving up the winding dirt road to the trailhead, we were startled to see scores of vehicles parked at the Caples Lake maintenance station: cars, trucks, horse trailers, and vans marked "Search and Rescue." Long tables set up in the maintenance yard held coffee urns and food, floodlight equipment, a PA system. Horses were tethered to bushes, and dogs lay panting in the shade of tall pines.

We learned what had happened. A child was lost. Kenny Miller, twelve years old and retarded, had been missing since the day before.

He'd been hiking with his parents and ten-year-old sister in Meiss Meadow. His dad was a high school teacher, his mom a speech therapist, like me. The parents and daughter had gone to look at something for a short while, leaving Kenny throwing stones in the stream. Kenny was out of their sight for three or four minutes. Then he was gone. Disappeared. No trace of him.

His parents looked and looked. They called other hikers in the meadow to search too. Eventually they contacted the forest service and reported him missing. Rescue teams assembled. One hundred and fifty people searched for him all night. Trained dogs tried to find his scent. Mounted rescue workers rode horses through thick pine forests.

Julian, Ben, and I parked the car at the trailhead and began the slow climb up switchbacks toward the ridge. The sky was gray and overcast, threatening rain. I remembered yesterday's storm: thunder and lightning crashing around us, hail stinging our faces, pellets of ice piling up in crannies of rocks along the trail.

Kenny Miller had also been out in that storm, wearing jeans, tennis shoes, and a white T-shirt. No jacket. He had the emotional and intellectual level of a four-year-old, his mother said. She couldn't predict how he'd act or what he might do.

Climbing the ridge, I searched for Kenny. I scanned the trail. I looked up the steep, rocky slope for a glimpse of him beside that rock, maybe, or off in those bushes. Maybe there in that stand of firs. A glimpse of his white shirt or tennis shoe sticking out from under a tree. Or the sight of his small figure curled near a boulder.

After a hard, sweaty climb, Julian, Ben, and I reached the top of the ridge, flopped on a rock, and gulped down our water. We hungrily ate lunch. I put on my parka against the cold wind. I kept watching for Kenny.

We looked down into Meiss Meadow, where Julian and I had been the year before, a lush paradise of mule ears, Indian paintbrush, lupine, and soft grass on the banks of meandering streams. Pine forests sloped up to high granite ridges ringing the meadow on three sides.

A small green helicopter flew low overhead, like a huge dragonfly. We heard the throbbing of its rotors as it flew back and forth. Then a twin-rotored army helicopter appeared over the ridge, also crisscrossing the meadow.

The late afternoon wind blew stronger. I zipped up my parka against the chill. As we descended the ridge I still looked for Kenny.

I thought of his mother, her anguish, her helplessness. I remembered three years ago when Julian got lost in the back country of Yosemite. We had hiked eight miles into Sunrise High Sierra Camp, and after supper Julian decided to stroll through the meadow at twilight. He wore only jeans and a T-shirt and carried no coat, no flashlight, no food. It had also hailed and snowed the night before. Darkness enveloped the camp and he hadn't returned. A ten-man search party went out to look for him.

"We'll search for one hour," the ranger said. "Then we'll have to wait till morning."

I felt sick to my stomach, fearing for the first time ever for Julian's life. I imagined his frozen body discovered stiff and lifeless under some tree. I sat on a rock and watched tiny dots of flashlights spread out into darkness. I heard the searchers calling "Julian . . . Julian."

They finally found him. He didn't have to spend the night alone in the wilderness without shelter. This happened one year before his Alzheimer's was diagnosed; looking back, I understood signs I didn't see then.

All this week while hiking, I guarded Julian closely. I had bought three whistles for our trip to the mountains, but Ben and Julian misplaced theirs after two days; only I wore my whistle. Julian often wandered off the trail. If he walked ahead of me, every few yards he would follow some worn track off to one side. Especially if the trail passed over rocks, he would lose it. How quickly he could wander out of sight around a boulder or outcropping and disappear.

How easily he could head off in one direction and I in another, until in only a few minutes miles could separate us. He could be walking into acres of wilderness thinking he would soon find the trail.

The next day, after climbing the ridge, we hiked to Shealor Lakes, east of Meiss Meadow. All day on the trail, I looked for Kenny. The newspaper said they had enough volunteers or I would have offered to help. I couldn't get Kenny out of my mind. He hadn't been found. Helicopters still flew low overhead, the dull throb of their rotors echoing up the canyon.

I imagined finding him.

"Kenny, Kenny," I'd say. "I know where your mom is. Come here, Kenny, have a sandwich. I'll take you to your mom." Should I give him my tuna sandwich first or should I give him water? Water first, I decided, then the sandwich. Should I stay with him and send Ben and Julian to run back to the search headquarters to say we'd found him—or should I go and they stay?

"I know where your mom is." I would reassure him. I would give him my coat. Often I imagined spotting his body, but I pushed that picture quickly away. Maybe I'd find him dead, like the hiker who did find him days later on the ridge near Steven's peak.

But I couldn't find Kenny Miller. I couldn't save him. I couldn't give him my sandwich or cover him with my coat.

Saying Goodbye to Stanford

Julian brought home his academic robe today from the Stanford Bookstore. He burst into our bedroom, where I lay resting on the bed in the hot afternoon before preparing dinner. The black mortarboard hat perched on his curly gray hair, tilted jauntily to one side. He threw the blue and gold satin hood over his shoulders, covering his T-shirt.

"I have the right colors because I got the gown in time this year," he said.

"Good going," I said, watching him admire his outfit in the mirror.

Julian usually forgot to pick up his gown until the last day before graduation, and then wore whatever colored hood they had left. Rarely did he wear the blue and gold of the University of California, where in 1958 he received his Ph.D.

Lying on the bed, watching Julian hang the black gown in his closet, I thought about Stanford's graduation this Sunday. It will be the last graduation procession he'll march in as a professor.

Next year, he will be on "early retirement"; he will officially be considered a professor emeritus.

Professor emeritus sounds so old, I thought. How did I come to be the wife of a professor emeritus? Professors emeriti are seventy or eighty. Julian is sixty-one; I'm fifty-four. Professor emeritus?

I wondered what thoughts would run through his head as he marched this last time as a professor? Would he feel as emotional as I did seeing him stand in our bedroom wearing his hat and hood? How would it feel to march into Frost Amphitheater on Sunday in the long double line of gowned and hooded academicians, his guild for twenty-nine years? When he retires next April on his sixty-second birthday, he will have been at Stanford for thirty years.

As Julian puttered about our bedroom, changing his clothes and sorting through papers, I lay thinking about our years at Stanford.

Julian came to the university in 1963 as a shy, tentative young assistant professor hired into the Physiology Department of the medical school three years after we were married. Ben, our first child, was nine months old. Julian taught physiology to medical students and mentored young scientists. He was awarded research grants (the first of many), and he investigated the influence of hormones on reproductive behavior. He wrote and published papers, soon earning tenure and promotion to Associate Professor, no small feat at Stanford University, whose medical school was fast becoming one of the best in the country.

Finally, after publishing scores of research papers in major physiology journals, speaking at national and international conferences, and becoming recognized as a leader in his field, he was promoted to professor, a well-deserved and hard-won honor. He progressed steadily along the steps in the academic pattern.

When Ben was three, our daughter Karen was born, and our son Jeff came along after that. The kids grew. I returned to Stanford to earn an M.A. in speech pathology and establish my career as a speech therapist. We both worked and raised our children; the years flew by. Now, here it was—June 1992, the last year of Julian's career.

Resting on my bed as the hot afternoon eased into evening, I looked back on our time at Stanford; floods of memories paraded before me.

Stanford housed us, fed us, supported us, and provided the framework for our lives. Stanford gave us a sabbatical at Oxford when Ben was seven, Karen four, and Jeff a baby. It sent Julian to a think tank in Seattle three years later. We spent another sabbatical in Athens, with a summer in a fishing village on Crete. A year in Washington, D.C., at the National Institutes of Health. These special years became markers for our lives, the dividing lines between periods: "We did this or that before Greece or after Oxford."

Sometimes I felt depressed over being uprooted from my life, work, and friends during these years away designed for his career and convenience. Often I felt jealous at the "power differential" between us. He went to an international conference in Rome or Tokyo, Sicily or Copenhagen, while I went to soccer games, Sunday school, and the supermarket. At times I was angry at Julian for not being more available. Yet, despite these shadows, Stanford sabbaticals added to the richness of our lives.

Lying in our bedroom in our house on the Stanford campus, I realized how academia has always been in the background: quarters beginning and ending, grant applications due and then their renewals, NIH study section reports, students and "postdocs" coming and going, along with the research associates who took their sabbaticals in Julian's lab.

I remembered how just after his last sabbatical in Washington, D.C., Julian first began worrying about his memory. Only he was aware of the problem, back then in 1986, nearly six years ago. Subtle changes: a little more time required to produce the name of a scientist or of the article or journal where a fact could be found. Lecture notes needed to be written in more detail. No more sparse one-page outlines from which he used to lecture spontaneously and well for an hour. More time needed to write a paper. Things he used to do rapidly and effortlessly began to require more time and concentration.

Characteristically, over many years, he had lost papers, double-scheduled appointments, arrived late, forgotten his wallet. He had always been an "absent-minded professor." His mother warned me when we married in 1960 that "Julian always loses his coats." He had been losing jackets since he was five. So in 1986 Julian quietly worried about the slow, insidious changes that, then, he alone could see.

A wave of sadness washed over me. I thought how now, June 1992, just two years after his diagnosis, all his professional knowledge had drained away. Cleaning out his desk and sorting through papers the other day, he read a chapter he wrote in a medical textbook and told me he didn't even know what it was about.

"Look at this paper," he said last night, handing me a reprint from the *Journal of Hormones and Behavior* entitled "Hormones and Sexual Behavior in Relationship to Aging in Male Rats."

"I don't have the slightest idea what this means," he said. The journal was dated 1992. My heart gave a thump. "You know," he confessed, "I can't even do arithmetic anymore. . . . I can't do any calculations."

For months I had known that Julian couldn't figure 15 percent for a restaurant tip and that he had trouble adding and subtracting numbers. He had trouble telling time. "Sixty-three," he said, for six-thirty, or "twenty-five" for two-fifty. He chunked the numbers into odd segments, putting any two adjacent numbers together.

From my bed I could see the black robe with velvet panels hanging in his closet next to his khaki trousers and colored shirts. The square mortarboard with the gold tassel lay on his dresser atop a messy pile of papers, the blue and gold satin hood draped over his desk.

I imagined the crowd next Sunday, mothers dressed in bright flowered dresses and wide-brimmed straw hats to shade their faces against the sun. Proud fathers photographing black-gowned sons and daughters. I heard the band playing "Hail Stanford, Hail," the song I had learned as a seventeen-year-old freshman in Roble Hall.

I envisioned the colorful procession, the long line of professors marching into the amphitheater, the blues, yellows, crimsons, greens, and whites of their academic hoods. Academia had been Julian's guild. Its values became his values, consciously and unconsciously, guiding and shaping his life. Pursuing new information, discovering how things work, consolidating what's known around a certain question, asking the next question, posing a new thesis that reconciles a conflict in the literature or explains some contradictory facts and thereby advances the field.

That's all behind him now, I thought. Julian can't do this any longer. He had imagined himself retired, sure, but not at this age. He had imagined himself doing research for years to come. And writing theoretical articles, maybe, or popular science.

I remembered his recent writings: phone messages for me. "Rosenne must coal as sown." I knew it meant "Call Roseanne as soon as possible." "Caul Hannah asks for a movew" meant "Call Hannah about going to a movie" and "The women who died about 6 months" meant "Call our friend whose husband died six months ago." I deciphered these quickly. I had spent twelve years working with children with language problems, and fortunately I've always loved guessing games.

Julian had set aside his academic career with grace. I realized that maybe I was being more nostalgic than he.

"I may not be intelligent anymore," he has told me on several occasions. "But I'm happy." I thought how he enjoys his life and likes what he's doing. He told me daily, "I'm a free and simple man."

Shadows inched across the loquat tree outside our bedroom window. It was nearly time to prepare dinner. The black gown hung where I could see it from my bed.

I thought of the fresh young faces of graduating seniors, conspicuous around the campus these June days, full of hope and promise, their lives wide open before them. They were celebrating the completion of an academic journey and marking the beginning of a new life ahead. For Julian and me, I thought, this commencement feels like an ending. It marks the end of his long, fruitful career and the end of our predictable life.

But I wondered if it could be a beginning of some sort for us too. Every closing of one door opens another. Setting down his academic obligations has freed Julian and given him space. To his credit, he was looking with joy and hopefulness at this commencement of his free and simple life.

I got up from the bed, closed Julian's closet door, and went to the kitchen to make dinner, feeling a rich mix of all that we had had, all that we were losing, and the big question mark of our life ahead.

"Who's the President?" Dr. M. Asked

"What's the date?" I asked my friend Louisa as she, two other women, and I began writing at Caffe Verona today. I wanted to put the date at the top of my page, and I couldn't remember what it was.

"June thirtieth," Louisa snapped back without hesitating.

"Of course," I thought. Being older than Louisa, sleepy this morning, and a little frazzled, I just needed a few seconds before coming up with the date. But I knew that we had returned from Silver Lake on June 26, that the Gay Pride Parade in San Francisco was June 28, and this was two days later. I could have figured it out.

Yesterday at Julian's yearly follow-up appointment with the neurologist, Dr. M. asked Julian the date. Julian didn't know. Silence. A long (excruciatingly painful) silence. Julian didn't say anything.

After a long pause he said, "June." He had managed to produce June. Then he said, "June ninth."

"It's more toward the end of June," said Dr. M. casually. "It's June twenty-ninth."

"Who's the president?" Dr. M. asked Julian as he knocked his knees with the little rubber hammer.

Julian sat on the examining table, his legs dangling over the edge. He wore beige cotton pants and a green T-shirt with a thin blue horizontal stripe. He kicked his legs back and forth, my big gray-haired, bearded kid.

I sat across the room in a chair, my head down, pretending to read cartoons in the *New Yorker.* I felt the way I had when I'd taken my children to the pediatrician for their annual checkups. They would sit up on the examining table bravely, alone, while I tried to melt into the background and let the pediatrician ask them questions.

"I don't like him, that fool!" Julian stalled for time. "That stupid guy. We've got to get him out of there. Bush," he said triumphantly. "Bush."

"Who's the vice president?" Dr. M. didn't let up. He slipped these questions into the conversation as he checked Julian's reflexes with the little hammer.

Julian's reflexes were great. His legs jerked forward after Dr. M. tapped his knees. Julian didn't answer about the vice president.

"Quayle," said Dr. M.

"Oh yeah, that stupid guy," Julian said.

"Remember what Quayle did recently, what mistake he just made that's been in the news?" Dr. M. tried to make it sound like a friendly chat instead of the mental status exam I knew it was.

Dr. M. had begun the appointment by asking Julian about his work, what his job was at Stanford, what his research was about. He sat back in his chair, stared intently at Julian, and studied him carefully. Julian answered in the most vague, rambling way. After that, Dr. M. started asking about the president and turned to me for information about the experimental drug, Tacrine, which Julian was taking.

At this time, June 1992, Tacrine was the only available drug for Alzheimer's, even though it showed only limited results in improving functioning in some mildly impaired patients. I had entered Julian in the clinical trial, desperate to do whatever I could to help him. Now the clinical trial had just ended.

Dr. M. and I discussed how to go about getting more Tacrine, which wasn't yet on the market. I told him I'd learned that only two physicians in the area had medical access to the drug. One, after saying two weeks ago that he would be glad to get it for Julian and that the drug company would probably pay for it, just phoned this morning to say he couldn't get it after all. I told Dr. M. I had called around all day trying to ensure that Julian could remain on the medication. Dr. M. listened, nodded, and said to let him know what transpired.

As the appointment ended, Dr. M. shook Julian's hand, said to call if any problems came up, and told us to come back in a year.

Sitting in Caffe Verona the next day, I remembered the vague dissatisfaction I had felt after the appointment. Dr. M. had been attentive. He had scrutinized Julian's behavior and listened carefully to his speech, assessing him as best he could. I knew I could call if medical problems developed, or if Julian needed a sedative or tranquilizer or antidepressant. I knew I could rely on him later.

But I felt somehow disappointed. It hadn't been a *bad* visit; it just hadn't felt helpful. I hadn't gotten anything from it. I had felt no sense of encouragement coming from him, had heard no remarks indicating he understood what a hard reality we lived with, no suggestions for how to manage or cope, no sense of compassion. If only he had said, "This is a difficult illness. Here are some ways to handle it. . . ." Or if he'd asked, "How are you both doing?" or "What things are troubling you now?"

I have already contacted the Alzheimer's Association, the Veteran's Hospital Alzheimer's and Memory Disorder Clinic, our local health library, the experimental drug trial. But I found all these resources myself; they weren't suggested by Julian's doctor. Maybe I was unrealistic in looking for support, reassurance, and guidance from a neurologist.

Sipping my latte, I wondered what Julian had experienced in that visit. We never discussed it. I imagined he had felt embarrassed over not being able to answer Dr. M.'s questions. Julian knows when he's covering up and not grasping what's going on. He has often told me that he hates feeling incompetant and losing face.

I remembered yesterday going to a coffee shop after Julian's appointment. Julian handed the cashier nine dollars even though she repeated "$5.25" three times; she looked at him with disgust. Later, when Julian and I returned to Stanford after coffee, he couldn't find the door of the medical school where his office is located. And he parked in the wrong parking lot near his old office. That night at home I found the missing lettuce in the freezer, black and crunchy, and the cleanser in the pot-and-pan cupboard.

Julian's increasing confusion scares me. Each discovery challenges me to accept him as he is, to accept his limitations. I cherish all the things we still do together, all the ways life is normal: walking to Printers Inc. for a cappuccino, sitting beside him on the couch watching a video, snuggling against his warm, familiar body under the sheets. This morning he brought me coffee in bed, as he has for years, and suddenly I treasured this gift which for decades I've taken for granted.

At Caffe Verona I looked up to see my three friends writing furiously in their notebooks. When I asked Louisa the date earlier, it had only momentarily slipped my mind. And in the doctor's office, though I paused myself before recalling Quayle's name, I could retrieve it.

I thought back to those few seconds when I had felt bewildered, puzzled, confused, that feeling of knowing what you want to say, but the words have escaped you. They are dangling there, elusive, out of reach. I magnified those feelings, extended and expanded them, not just to the date, but to names, words, locations of objects . . . all day long, day after day, hour after hour, a fuzzy slowness that won't go away—a frightening glimpse of what life must be like for Julian. How does it feel to really not remember?

The Alzheimer's Couples' Group

In the Alzheimer's Couples' Group yesterday, I slipped quietly into a seat. Two psychiatric nurses and ten couples settled into a large circle in a conference room at the Veteran's Hospital.

Looking around, I could hardly tell which person had Alzheimer's and which was the spouse. Well-dressed couples sat on blue chairs, most of them in their seventies, I guessed. I was fifty-three, the youngest by ten years at least. After attending six sessions, Julian had stopped coming. He didn't like it and I agreed it wasn't helping him then. I was alone this month, unclear why, exactly, I came.

What was I doing here, I asked myself, just as I had at each monthly meeting. Entering a room full of Alzheimer's patients was frightening. I wasn't the facilitator, as I was at Parents and Friends of Lesbians and Gays, where the fact that Ben was gay was no longer a problem. Julian had Alzheimer's—and I was a person needing help.

Waiting for the session to start, I checked out faces. One woman and two men had a subtle look I recognized, a sort of glazed, bewildered blankness in their eyes, a slightly hunched posture, a mild shuffling gait.

But most looked fine, the men attractive, nicely dressed. You might see them on a golf course, in a restaurant or shopping center.

The psychiatric nurse, Helen, a petite dark-haired woman in a purple blazer, opened the meeting. "How are you?" she asked, looking around the room. "What's been happening?"

"Frank won't sleep at night," one woman answered. "It's two A.M. and I can't get him to bed. I'm afraid to sleep myself for fear he'll go outside or turn on the stove."

"Sam's been aggressively attacking our grandson," said another.

"Ted can't dress himself any longer. He puts underwear on over his trousers."

After each woman spoke, Helen offered suggestions. In a calm, gentle voice, she explained what might be causing the new behavior and how caregivers might respond. Everyone listened intently. A few took notes.

In yesterday's meeting only spouses spoke. The Alzheimer's patients said nothing, except for one thin, gray-haired woman, who smiled and made irrelevant comments. A year ago, when Julian and I first went to the group, everyone had introduced themselves and made appropriate remarks. But they had changed over the year.

A lean, muscular man named Arthur struggled to speak.

"Ba ... ba ... ba ...," he stammered. "Di-bika, di-bika, di-bika ..."

Arthur's wife held his hand. She whispered, "We're going home soon, Arthur," or "We'll leave when the meeting's over."

"Di-bika, di-bika," he said.

Arthur got up and walked out the door seven times in fifteen minutes. The second nurse followed him into the hall so that his wife could get some relief. Arthur paced up and down, as if search-ing for something. He wandered restlessly about the room, sitting in one chair, then another, always returning to his wife. He sat next to her for a few minutes, staring as if wanting to speak, but only his dreadful gibberish emerged. His wife laid her hand on his shoulder and rubbed his back.

Arthur returned to his chair after each little foray, as a tod-dler scrambles away from Mother to explore the unknown and then returns for a pat, a touch, some contact that says "I'm here. You're not alone. You're okay."

"We're going home soon, Arthur," she said, like a gray-haired mom quieting a huge two-year-old.

"He paces all day long," his wife said, trying to focus on the discussion. "He can't concentrate on anything."

My heart went out to her. How could she stand this? How could she bear it? How did she maintain her life and sanity living with Arthur? Day after day, alone with him. He was once an intel-ligent man, her husband, her companion. They once shared ideas and thoughts; they'd made love, plans, and dinner together.

Watching Arthur, hyperbolic phrases popped into my head: "destroyer of the mind, annihilator of the self, obliterator of the soul", words I'd read in articles about Alzheimer's, journalists' descriptions of later stages. "Quit obsessing on those phrases," I warned myself. "They don't help me now with Julian."

I needed to focus on our present reality, not sink into despair imagining the future. I couldn't bear to think of Julian like Arthur. I wanted to find Julian's strengths and relate to all the ways in which he was normal, instead of sliding into clutching fear, that black hopelessness which sometimes enveloped me.

The group discussion turned to day care. Most of the men went to a senior day program, and wives discussed their husbands' adjustment, in the same way my daughter and her friends dis-cussed toddlers' preschools. They stated why this or that program was or wasn't appropriate and which provided buses. I listened, stiff and uncomfortable, glad Julian wasn't there, resisting believ-ing these problems might one day be ours.

"I have simple puzzles for Sam," said one woman. "Six or ten pieces. I put them on the breakfast table in the morning and that keeps him busy while I drink my coffee and read the paper." Sam sat silently beside her, a tall, handsome man, white hair framing a tan face; he wore a smart black and white sweater, and looked like someone you would find behind a mahogany desk in his office.

"I give Jack buttons to sort," said another cheerily. "I tell him to put them in separate jars." This woman organized outings for the Alzheimer's Social Club the group has started. How could she be so cheerful, I thought, trying to picture Julian and me at an Alzheimer's dinner dance.

"You can give them pennies to count," said another. "They can wrap pennies in piles of ten."

My heart sank. Would Julian one day be doing puzzles, sorting buttons, and counting pennies? Only two years ago he was a professor at Stanford Medical School. He wrote grants, published papers in journals, and administered a major research program at this V.A. hospital where the Alzheimer's group met. Julian and I discussed books, movies, politics in Israel. He helped edit my writing. He was my confidant and best friend; we traveled, hiked, and skied together. Would Julian one day go to day care?

I looked around the room at the faces of all these brave women, imagining what they dealt with daily. My complaints seemed petty next to theirs. Julian still ran his own life, sort of. He could stay alone, for an evening, several days even, though I was already uneasy about that. He was the only man not in day care.

But these women lived through it. They showed me courage, loyalty, resilience, and love. These wives did everything: running their households on top of caring for handicapped mates. Their lives were restricted; they couldn't leave home without finding a sitter. Each watched loved companions grow backward into retarded children.

One said her husband got lost for seventeen hours just blocks from their house. He couldn't remember how to phone home. Even though he could still play two sets of tennis, he went to adult day care with frail folks in wheelchairs and walkers.

I had seen a photo of him at the Center: a bright-looking man in a corduroy jacket at a lunch table surrounded by elderly ladies in flowered dresses. He should have been at Lockheed designing aerospace equipment, or backpacking in the Sierra, or traveling to France. Not senior day care at sixty-three!

The group's talk turned to difficult weekends.

"I end up screaming at him," one woman confessed.

"All caregivers of demented patients yell," Helen reassured us. "It's okay to let out that stress."

"On weekends there's no separation," another explained, her eyes misting over. "We're alone together for two long, unstructured days. I feel terrible after I yell. But the bottom line is that I love him."

The pluckiness of these women amazed me. How ingenious they were at accommodating to continual change, determined to keep their lives going, relentless, like this disease, in figuring out new ways to handle ever-shifting, chaotic scenes. They gave me glimpses of how I might cope.

One arranged for a psychology student to live in a spare bedroom and help care for her husband in exchange for rent. One tried four day care centers before finding one her husband liked. One planned a vacation with her sister and brother-in-law so that she could have relief, company, and fun. Another took her husband to a respite house and traveled to Hawaii for the first time alone.

But Julian hadn't reached the stages their husbands were at. Maybe he never would. All Alzheimer's patients are different; the disease progresses at different rates. Some decline rapidly and some decline slowly; some have long, stable plateaus where deterioration seems to stop. It's impossible to predict what will happen to an individual, Helen told me. Uncertainty made it difficult to plan. Maybe Julian would die from a heart attack before speaking gibberish or needing day care. Yet did I really wish that?

"I'm not like them," Julian told me after each group session. "I'll never be like that. I'm healthy and strong. I have a deep feeling I'm okay."

As Julian and I hovered together at the brink of change, the Alzheimer's pamphlet's sentence persisted: ". . . relentless, progressive deterioration . . . until eventually patients will be unable to communicate and will require total care." The words I couldn't get out of my brain.

Helen announced that the session was over. Looking at my watch, I saw ninety minutes had passed. As couples chatted over coffee and cookies, I slipped quickly out the door, my head throbbing, feeling drained and exhausted.

The next day I met a friend for lunch. Her husband had died four months earlier in a nursing home for Alzheimer's patients. He too had taught at Stanford. She had kept him home under "twenty-four-hour surveillance" for half a year before she could no longer manage and finally placed him in residential care.

"I ran a locked facility for six months," she told me over our chicken salads.

We discussed his last years, last months, last weeks, and last days, and I listened with a heavy, compassionate heart. I held her hand. After lunch, as we prepared to go our separate ways, she hugged me and said simply, "Love your man. Go out now and enjoy your life."

I knew, at this stage, that was exactly what I needed to do.

Preparing for Silence

Last night Julian and I ate *arroz con pollo* in my friend Connie's patio from blue-green French plates on a woven tablecloth surrounded by flowering jasmine. Connie's daughter was there, and her tenant, and Paul and Dorothea and Dorothea's sister who's visiting from Canada. Comfortable, pleasant, easy talk, or so I thought.

But afterward, when we were home in bed, Julian cried. He cried because I was impatient with him. It happened so fast.

I lay in bed reading the Sunday *Examiner*, relaxing a little before turning out the light. Julian walked around in his pajamas, shuffling papers. He asked me something and interrupted my reading. Every time I read a sentence, he asked me another question and I had to reread the sentence. No big deal, perhaps, but there was more to it than that. I couldn't understand what he was saying. I couldn't get it without stopping and focusing totally on what he said.

While I was trying to read, he began telling about a letter he had received from a doctor in Spain. He needed to respond and couldn't do it alone. I wasn't sure what he wanted. So I snapped out an answer. Maybe I sucked in my breath loudly. Suddenly he was crying.

He jumped up from the bed, went to the bathroom, and brushed his teeth. From the bathroom I heard funny sounds, half laugh, half cry, an odd choked-off sob. Julian rarely cries. And even then, not for long.

"Come to bed, Julian," I said. "I'm sorry. I didn't mean to hurt your feelings." I apologize a lot now, I realized, because often I can't control what I say.

Listening to his snuffling noises in the bathroom, I thought of Arthur. Compared to Arthur, Julian was a brilliant speaker; compared to others in the Alzheimer's group, an articulate companion. I was filled with shame.

Julian returned and lay on his side of the bed, his back to me. I heard more choked sobs. I rolled over and tried to hold him, to cradle his head on my chest, to stroke him. But he was tight and locked up.

"It's sad, Julian. It's okay to cry." I encouraged him to let go, to allow himself to experience what he was feeling. But he didn't want to. He sat up woodenly in a cross-legged meditation pose, closed his eyes, and blocked me out. Meditating didn't work. After a minute he slid down into my arms.

"It's not your fault," he said. "It's me. You don't want to listen. You don't want to talk to me. I don't blame you. No one wants to talk to me."

I wrapped my arms around him and hugged him tight.

"But when you do that, it's like you're laughing at a sick person," he said. He meant my hissing response to his request to help him with the letter.

"You're right." I said again, "I'm sorry."

"I felt so bad tonight at Connie's dinner," he said. "I just sat there. I couldn't talk. I felt uncomfortable and didn't know what to say."

He wasn't used to being a quiet person. He was used to being witty, quick, sarcastic, enjoying fast, clever repartee.

Again I named the quiet people we knew. I reminded him that at any dinner table, there are people who don't talk much. He could sit and listen and still be part of the group.

"Speak to someone next to you," I told him. "Talk with just one person. It's too hard to join in fast group talk." Julian was becoming increasingly self-conscious in groups, which we'd discussed countless times before.

At breakfast the next morning, I realized our old easy talk was gone, remarks exchanged while dressing or undressing, while making coffee and putting bagels on the table, while doing dishes or folding laundry. Julian can't talk and do something else at the same time anymore—this man who used to do six things at once.

I see, too, that I can't understand Julian if I'm doing something else. I have to stop and listen. I need to focus on what he's saying, give full attention. I must decode awkward phrases to get his message. I must unscramble jumbled sentences to find the meaning. I guess at what he wants to say when he can't finish a sentence or when he produces the opposite word or a word oddly related to the one he means.

Sipping my coffee, I remembered how for years Julian had flirted with meditation. Off and on, he went to retreats, read, and listened to tapes. Meditation appealed to him long ago, then as a quieting of his highly verbal, chattering mind. Now it offers a way of being silent without fear.

"Maybe I'll be a hermit," he joked with me recently. "I'll grow my beard and go live in a cave."

"Not a bad idea," I'd said. "I'll live in the valley and bring you food."

Once, while driving home from the Alzheimer's couples' group, we talked about his trouble speaking. "It's okay," he said, "as long as I have you to talk to."

Remembering the exchange, the responsibility of this role hit me. I'll need more patience than I have now. I'll need to learn what's so infuriating to me about Julian's speech. In all my years as a speech therapist, I never fully appreciated the frustrations of the parents whose children I taught. What is it exactly that's so terrible?

It's not that one garbled exchange is so difficult. Rather, it's the loss of comfortable sharing. Each miscommunication drives the wedge of separation in a little deeper. It widens the gap between who Julian is now and who he used to be, between what could have been and all we've lost.

I realized that our tangled talks are emotionally loaded, far beyond the content of what's being discussed. They remind me of the past—wisdom, knowledge, intimacy, problem solving, joking— gone. Not yet gone, maybe, but fast disappearing. They also bring up fear of the future: a time when Julian may not be able to talk at all, may be unresponsive and mute, his biggest fear. And mine.

In the car last Friday, he had opened up to that fear. "I'm beginning to imagine," he said, "how it feels to be someone who can't talk.

"But my soul is still me," he said. "I'm still myself. In a few years, though, I may not be able to speak."

Sitting at the kitchen table, I remembered back to a recent dinner at another friend's house. Someone spoke of meeting a sixty-five-year-old man in India about to go into retreat and take a vow of silence. He was "preparing for silence." I wondered what he was doing to "prepare" and wished I'd asked. But the phrase stuck with me.

Maybe that's what Julian and I were doing now, each in our own ways: preparing for his silence.

I'm Too Often Furious

"Gramma, I doed dishes." Celina called me on the phone today. "And I goed to the park."

My grandaughter is two and a half, that fabulous age when language bursts forth. Speech now reveals her thoughts. Her ideas transform into sounds, sounds link into words, words combine into phrases, phrases bloom into sentences . . . transmitted across air into the ear and mind of another: the miracle of speech.

Everyday Celina acquires new vocabulary, while daily more words slip away from Julian. He tries to hang on to them, but Alzheimer's tangles and neural plaques steal his precious words. He makes lists—stores, food, restaurants, clothes. If he struggles for a word and finally remembers it, he writes it down. Periodically he reads the lists, hoping to hang on to words a little longer.

On the big oak desk in his study sit a red thesaurus and a Webster's dictionary. "I'll read the dictionary every day," he says. "It's sad to lose so many beautiful words. . . ."

"Write me names," Julian says. "I want you to write down all the names. Everyone's names." He's been asking me to do this for weeks. And it's true that names are going fast.

"I'll make a list," I've promised. "We'll have categories— friends, family, professional colleagues." That may help . . . for a while.

At a phenomenal rate Celina acquires language. Her word combinations are getting longer. She uses pronouns, plurals, verb endings, and irregular verb forms.

At the same time, Julian's language is breaking down. He confuses pronouns: "he" for "she," "him" for "her," "them" for "us." He often says the opposite of what he means: "salt" for "pepper," "go" for "come," "up" for "down," "buy" for "sell." He misuses words: "library" for "bookstore," "hour" for "day," "minute" for "second," "bus" for "car." He uses long, vague circumlocutions when he can't come up with the desired word: "You know, the big thing that goes up from the main place" for "University Avenue." Or, "That piece of paper where you write on it how much and they give you money" for "check."

Sometimes he overgeneralizes irregular past tense verbs. "I writed . . ." he said the other day, just like Celina.

When Celina says "writed," it's normal for her. "Gramma, I writed a letter," she says. Or, "I drinked juice." That's how children acquire grammatical forms. They miraculously learn linguistic "rules" in some mysterious way. Two-year-olds perceive patterns: past tense verb forms add "ed." Then they overgeneralize regular past tense rules to irregular forms—"writed," "goed," "doed," "eated," "drinked." Language is not learned by imitation alone; it's acquired by the mysterious perception of linguistic patterns. Later children learn the irregular forms—"wrote," "went," "ate," "drank."

Not only does Julian have difficulties finding words, the problem he's most aware of, but his syntax is becoming garbled too. Compared to many Alzheimer's patients at a mild–moderate stage, Julian's language is especially impaired. Some people retain good syntax even at more advanced stages, though their language doesn't make sense. Julian knows what he wants to say; he just can't say it.

It's also getting harder for him to write, this articulate man who prided himself on his accurate use of words, his meticulous choice of the right word with the exact nuance. As a scientist he wrote clearly. Colleagues quoted his chapters and requested reprints because he summarized, clarified, and assimilated difficult material.

Julian spent his youth in the Glasgow public library, skipping school as a boy and spending hours reading everything he could lay his hands on: Marx, Freud, Oscar Wilde, E. M. Forster, and an obscure Russian anarchist named Pyotr Alekseyevich Kropotkin.

Now he can barely write a correct sentence. He scribbles illegible notes in his calendar, which later even he can't read. Or he adds a garbled line at the end of my letters.

A speech therapist reporting on Julian would describe his language as deteriorating due to a primary progressive dementia. He displays both comprehension and production problems secondary to progressive brain disease. He has aphasiclike deficits in word finding, fluency, syntax, comprehension, auditory processing, and discrimination.

Julian sums it up simply: "Bloody Alzheimer's stealing my words!"

Ironic that I spent twelve years as a speech pathologist working with neurologically impaired children with language problems. I remember a red-haired, freckle-faced five-year-old I taught for years. I tape-recorded language samples of Eric's speech. For hours I analyzed his word combinations to see which grammatical constructions were present and which were missing. I devised games to model and teach use of specific structures that should have been present. I consulted with his parents.

Am I therefore more understanding of Julian's language problems?

Absolutely not! Try as I might to remain considerate, I am too often furious at his mistakes. It's unfair to him when I get angry, I know. But frustration floods over me when I can't understand him or he misunderstands me. Working as a speech therapist has not prepared me to be patient; I am only excruciatingly sensitive to his mistakes.

When Celina says, "I goed there," I marvel at the miracle of her speech. When Julian says, "I eated cake," his words jab like hot pokers into my heart.

A Wise Man Speaks

Grabbing the Walkman and sliding the earphones over my head, I dash out the door for my morning walk. Cool air brushes my face. The sky is overcast and foggy, the silver sun hidden behind gray clouds. I stride up the path lined by honey-colored grasses. No one's in sight. My head buzzes: Call the carpet company. Return three hotline calls. Leave a check for the cleaners. Unlock the front door. Write a note to the tenant. Buy lettuce, toilet paper, and milk.

I punch the Play button on the Walkman. I don't even know what tape is in there. Thich Nhat Hanh, a Vietnamese Buddhist, begins to speak. Julian bought this tape several weeks ago and has been listening to it at night in bed. How fitting that this tape should be in the Walkman today.

"We must remember four things," Thich Nhat Hanh says. "It is in our nature to grow old. It is in our nature to get sick. It is in our nature to be separated from loved ones. It is in our nature to die." His voice is gentle, calm, and soothing. Somehow it isn't frightening to hear these words.

The path leads me past the school where all three of my children went. The climbing equipment stands empty, the playground deserted. In an hour the orange and blue plastic tunnels, tubes, slides and platforms will be swarming with children. Now they sit like a huge hamster maze you'd see at a pet shop.

Twenty years ago, when my children played here, the climbing equipment consisted of gray metal bars, a slide, and a swing set. My children are young adults now, the age I was when we moved to our house on the Stanford campus and my kids attended this school. My daughter has small children of her own, and I bring my grandchildren to climb on the blue and orange plastic tunnels.

Thich Nhat Hanh speaks about growing old. "It is in our nature to grow old," he repeats. Julian is growing old. So am I. Julian's hair is gray now. I hardly remember his brown, wavy hair and thick, dark beard, and I'm shocked when I see them in photos.

As I stride along the path past my children's school, I am calmed by Thich Nhat Hanh's words; I take them in deeply and they soothe me. But then a wave of awareness of losing Julian overwhelms me, and the words feel like trite clichés, of no use whatsoever to lessen my grief.

"It is in our nature to lose our loved ones," Thich Nhat Hanh continues. "There's no escaping it."

"Yes," I think, "but not now. I'm too young for all this. Not me. Not Julian. Not yet!" But if not now, then it will come later. Illness just came earlier to us than expected, but the issues of illness are the same.

Julian's body bends over sometimes these days, and he sort of shuffles. He limps now, arthritis in his feet. His muscles are less firm and his arms midway between my eighty-one-year-old father's frail arms and the powerful arms of our son Ben. Sometimes Julian falls asleep on the sofa while we're reading or watching television. His glasses slip down his nose and his mouth falls open.

When this happens, I feel abandoned, inch by inch, in slow motion. I know I must learn to do things with him, yet enjoy them by myself. I must let him take what he can from an experience, but not let my enjoyment depend on sharing it with him.

I leave the school, turn the corner and pass tall white-barked eucalyptus trees. Their trunks feel smooth and cold to my touch; their leaves fill the air with a pungent, sweet smell.

Summer 1992

"It is in our nature to be ill," Thich Nhat Hanh says again. If I expect Julian and me to always be healthy, then when illness comes, I think something is wrong. This is *not* how it's supposed to be! I feel attacked, violated, enraged, ashamed. But if illness *is* how it's supposed to be, how it just is sometimes, then I can feel more accepting. Well, maybe . . .

Out here, in the early morning air, quiet, alone on this path surrounded by eucalyptus and oaks, dried grasses and rock roses, I glimpse acceptance. My cancer and Julian's Alzheimer's are *our* diseases. They are what has come to us—no one knows why. They are what we've been given to handle, the cards we've been dealt. Not blindness or deafness, not kidney or heart disease, not stroke or diabetes or cerebral palsy or Parkinson's or multiple sclerosis . . . the list of diseases goes on forever.

We don't have those other diseases. We have our diseases. We're the same as other folks with illness, only the illnesses are different. I feel a great connection to all others who endure.

There's a river of pain, sorrow, fear, and suffering that runs deep beneath us. It's simply there, a powerful current running below our surface life. As we journey through life we periodically tap down into it and feel "the pain," as Stephen Levine puts it. We get in touch with those age-old existential questions: the meaning of loss, abandonment, separation, and death. Often these days I feel the pain of growing old, becoming ill, and losing my loved ones.

Yet, Thich Nhat Hanh says that "anguish and suffering come from not understanding that these things *are* in our nature." Can I learn not to fear experiencing my cancer and Julian's Alzheimer's? Can I learn not to panic over the thought of losing Julian? Can I learn to let go of anguish? Can I learn to accept being ill and alone? Can I learn to be at ease with dis-ease?

I'm turning the corner and heading back to my street. Cars move along the road, folks driving to work. Children walk to school now and climb into the plastic tunnels. Back home in our courtyard, I switch off the Walkman. In the kitchen the clock over the stove reads "7:45."

Julian stands by the sink in his khaki shorts and blue T-shirt fumbling with the coffeepot, trying to make coffee. He smiles and strips off his shirt. His chest glistens with sweat—he's just returned from his morning run. His chest looks hard, firm, familiar.

"Where's that coffee thing that goes on the top of that other thing where you pour it into?" he asks.

"You mean the filter?" I ask, handing it to him. The filter was on the countertop right in front of him, but so many other objects cluttered the counter that he couldn't see it. It's getting harder for Julian to scan an array of objects and select one he wants. More and more he is confused by visual clutter.

I pull off my earphones and stash the tape recorder back in the cupboard. Julian brings two brightly painted mugs to the table. We sit down to hot coffee, granola, yoghurt, and strawberries. The strawberries are large and juicy, fresh from Webb Ranch, and when I bite into each one, it bursts open and fills my mouth with sweetness.

Exquisitely Balanced

Dinner last night at our friend Hannah's was pleasant. Hannah, her daughter, Julian, and I ate in her garden on a picnic table: chicken, corn on the cob, eggplant, squash, and a green salad.

Afterwards Julian, Hannah, and I walked for an hour by the bay, past shiny, dark blue ponds, past grassy marshes where ducks and pelicans and terns dove into the water to feed on twilight suppers. The red ball of the setting sun turned honey-colored grass to gold, deepened the blue of the ponds, and made the marsh glow. Snowy egrets stood motionless: thin white lines against the gold.

We walked and talked—easy light chatter—about mutual friends and work. When we returned to Hannah's house, we sat around the cluttered kitchen table eating ice cream and fresh blueberries. Hannah's kids hung out in the kitchen, refilling their bowls, talking about exams and arguing over who should do the dishes. A homey, comfortable evening.

Driving home, I asked Julian whether there was a VCR in his lab so that his secretary could start typing his autobiography tapes. The first two came last week and we'll get another tomorrow. Julian has started meeting with a psychology student who will videotape a twelve-session "life review."

But Julian didn't understand what I was saying. I rephrased the question and then repeated it. I tried shorter questions. I tried simple statements building to the essential part. I wasn't getting through. He made irrelevant comments. The conversation went around in circles, getting nowhere.

"What's a VCR?" he finally asked.

I began again. "Remember we got two videotapes from Susan last week? Tapes of your autobiography? Remember watching the tapes? When your secretary transcribes them, she'll need a television and a VCR. Is there a VCR in your lab?" I didn't know how to explain it more clearly.

My heart sank. I felt cold. I felt myself drawing in and closing off from Julian. I wanted to go away. It was so hard to talk to him, so painful when he didn't get it. What was the point of trying to talk or explain things? The pleasant evening with Hannah ended on this blue note as I pulled into our driveway.

Switching off the ignition, I grabbed my purse and walked quickly into the house, leaving Julian sitting motionless in the car. He sat forlornly in the passenger seat and didn't get out. I turned on lights and switched on the ten o'clock news. As I put on my pajamas I realized that I must keep talking to Julian. I must continue including him and pretending life is "normal." I mustn't withdraw. I mustn't quarrel with him or express irritation. Yet I felt such despair.

Julian came into the bedroom.

"Come. Let's watch the Democratic convention on the news," I said quietly, patting the bed beside me, trying to salvage the evening. He didn't respond.

Soon Ben arrived home from work and asked about dinner with Hannah. I told him about our walk in the sunset. Julian, Ben, and I watched the news together: A man and woman with AIDS eloquently pleaded for more government funding. Jesse Jackson addressed the convention, Jimmy Carter spoke, and so did a lesbian supervisor from San Francisco.

After the news Julian switched off the light. He rolled over to his side of the bed and turned his back to me. I wanted to sink into sleep. I had no energy to undo the coldness and distance that had descended. All I could muster was the energy to reach out, touch his shoulder, and ruffle his hair in the darkness.

"G'night, darling," I said. "See you in the morning." I tried to make my voice casual and loving, as if nothing were wrong, but I couldn't sleep.

This garbled exchange, like countless others, drove me away from Julian. I felt so alone. Gone were spontaneous talks, our old intimate sharing. I realized I was talking less and less about anything important and that a wedge of silence was growing between us.

I still habitually chattered on and told him things about my day. I remembered returning from my writer's group last week, for instance, telling him Maureen and Henri's good news about being accepted to a poetry conference at Squaw Valley. Simple enough, I thought.

But then I had to explain who Maureen was, and Henri, and where was Squaw Valley. And no, it wasn't me who was going, and no, I'm going away in mid-September to the mountains, and we're going to Seattle together over Labor Day, and all that is happening after his brother and sister-in-law visit in July . . . and by then I'm sorry I ever brought up the subject of Maureen and Henri, because he never got the point of what I tried to tell him in the first place.

"I'm lonely," I'd told Ben earlier in the kitchen, even though Julian is still very much here.

Lying in bed next to a now-sleeping Julian, I thought of my sisters-in-law Jenny and Claire: Their husbands are dead. Gone completely. Shrouded in cold graves. How they must long for the contact I still have with Julian. I thought of our friends Hannah and Penny, both widows, younger than I, their husbands lost to cancer.

Wouldn't Claire or Jenny, Penny or Hannah, give anything to have back Terry and Sam, Jay and Larry, as I have Julian? He is still here, warm and comforting in my bed, coming home each night for dinner, a swim, a walk, a concert, a movie, a cuddle.

Lying quietly in the dark, I suddenly understood my balancing act. I must balance the reality of present life with Julian against my awareness of greater losses to come. I saw myself poised on a seesaw. When I sink slightly, I must do something to regain equilibrium. Now down, now back up. Each time I drop to one side, I must adjust my mood or self-statements to regain balance.

My side of the bed felt lonely and cheerless. I rolled over, across the cold space between Julian's body and mine, spooned myself around his warm back, and fell into warm, familiar sleep.

Julian's Worries

Julian's therapist, Susan, just came to the clinic lobby to get him for the fourth session of his "life review." She handed me the tape of their previous meeting. We had agreed that Julian would have twelve videotaped sessions talking about his life in a structured way. When she and Julian left, I took out my journal, settled into the brown armchair, and began to write.

I remembered last week at home, when Julian and I watched the first two tapes. The first scene showed Julian sitting in a leather recliner in the therapy room, listening to Susan explain what they would do.

"We're on an adventure together," she said simply. "Neither of us has done this before. We're exploring."

"I'd like to do two things here," Susan said. "First, this is a time for you to say whatever's on your mind. Second, we'll go over your life story in five-year intervals. We'll tape each session and you can use the tapes for your autobiography."

In the first five minutes, out tumbled Julian's worries about his poor memory, his language problems, and his failing brain. He couldn't find the right words, he said. He didn't need to tell her. He struggled constantly as he spoke: pausing, stopping midsentence, putting his head in his hands.

"Thoughts just fly away. I have a great idea and it disappears. I can hardly write," he told Susan. "I think of something I want to say, but I can't remember the words. I go to the dictionary to try to find a word or look up spelling. By then, the thought's gone. It goes like this all day."

"It must be so hard for you," Susan said, out of sight of the camera, which focused only on Julian. She never appeared on the tape. I only heard her comforting voice.

In my initial meeting with Susan, I explained why I had come. I had heard a lecture on how reminiscence can help Alzheimer's patients. The lecturer spoke of psychological life stages, the last one involving the need to make sense of your life.

I told Susan that Julian had started his autobiography when he first noticed his memory problems. As his career faded he began writing a memoir, and when people asked what he was doing last year on his sabbatical, he told them proudly, "Working on my autobiography."

"Great idea," friends said.

"His project has layers of meaning," I told her.

Life kept its usual form. He went each morning to the library and quietly wrote. He gave handwritten drafts to his secretary, who typed them into the computer and returned clean copy. Then he edited the manuscripts, scratching out words and moving sentences: the familiar process of his long writing career.

I explained to Susan that it was now much harder. Julian would sit in his study for hours and produce one short paragraph with misspelled words, ungrammatical sentences and phrases in illogical order. He had trouble sequencing ideas. Thoughts flew out of his head before he could write them; sometimes one might return, other times not. Gone, too, was his sophisticated language, his original way of saying things.

"Don't worry about being clever," I told him. "Just get the ideas down . . ."

We both knew the unstated end of that sentence: ". . . before you forget."

I told Susan that Julian first hoped his memoir would be beautifully written, perhaps even published. But it soon became obvious this wasn't to be.

"Aim it at our children and grandchildren," I urged Julian as time went on. "Tell the kids stories from your life."

"Forget about writing beautifully," I repeated. "Just get it down."

Seeing Julian's struggle, I brought out the tape recorder. We taped conversations about his childhood in Scotland, his adolescence in the Jewish youth movement in England, and his years in Israel in the early fifties. I transcribed the tapes and handed him interviews to edit.

"But it's not *interesting*," he complained. "This is just *talking*. Not good writing."

"Work with it," I urged him. "Cut out repetitions. Make the language better. Go slow. You have time."

Julian's satisfaction waxed and waned. One day he was enthusiastic and appreciative of my help, the next day impatient and despairing over the gap between what was on paper and what he had hoped it would be.

On his birthday this year, I told Susan, he came home long-faced.

"It's no good. I can't write." He threw papers on the table. "I can't do it."

"I'll help you edit them," I said. "Ben will help you. Don't stop. They're important."

About this time, I had heard the lecture on reminiscence. I wanted to help Julian with his autobiography, but I couldn't write his story on top of everything else I had to do. I explained all this the first time Susan and I met.

I remembered the end of the first tape, when they talked about Julian's childhood in Glasgow. He related a favorite story: nearly choking to death at his circumcision. His parents gave eight-day-old baby Julian sponge cake soaked in wine at his *bris* and he choked on crumbs.

On the second tape Julian described his best friend, a boy named Chaim. Julian and Chaim were inseparable buddies for years. They wrote plays, argued politics, hung out in the public library, and cut school together.

"Doesn't Chaim mean 'life'?" Susan asked. "Chaim was exciting. He brought you energy and life."

Tears spilled down my cheeks as I watched those tapes. Susan was helping Julian structure his thoughts and make sense of things. She found threads of meaning in his rambling anecdotes and knit them together. She spoke gently, but mostly she listened. Julian had an ally, someone to hear him and appreciate him . . . someone else besides me.

Excited, I phoned Susan the next day to tell her I had seen the tapes and was so happy.

"I really like Julian," she answered. "He is such a sweet man."

"You're patient with him," I said. "And you speak clearly."

"Well, it's not easy to find the right level, but I'm learning. It must be so difficult for you." Her voice softened. She told me she felt privileged to be involved in our project.

"Julian's confused about why he is coming," I told Susan. "He likes talking to you and feels good when he leaves. But he keeps saying, 'I didn't learn anything. I know everything already.'"

I explained over and over that Susan was helping him write his autobiography. He was confusing her sessions with the experimental support group he had gone to a year ago in San Francisco and with the couples' group we used to attend.

"When Julian came home after the second meeting, he wanted to quit," I told her. "He couldn't remember why he was there. But after the last time, he was delighted. Whatever happened was good."

"I'm glad you like what's going on," she said. "I'll try to explain to Julian again clearly."

Sitting in the lobby writing in my journal, I realized Susan was providing exactly what I wanted: structured sessions of "life review." Not only did she question Julian systematically, she found themes and connections. And she encouraged him to talk about present fears.

Curling my legs in the brown chair, I gave a long sigh. Julian had someone to talk to besides me.

But something else was happening in these sessions with Susan, and in my journal writings as well. I didn't know what exactly, but for both Julian and me, transforming feelings into words and putting memories onto paper seemed crucial. Out of decline, something was emerging.

Summer 1992

Susan and Julian were returning now. I heard them laughing and talking as they walked down the hall, Julian's hour of life review over and my hour of writing too. As they entered the lobby, I stuck the top on my pen, closed my journal, and stood to greet them.

I *Share* My *Fears*

Driving along the curving road, I glanced at Julian beside me in the car. He gazed out the window at brown hills studded with eucalyptus and live oak and whistled a Yiddish tune. We had hastily thrown bathing suits, clean shirts, massage oil, and books into duffel bags and headed for the beach for a night away. It was our anniversary; we'd been married thirty-two years. I began humming the tune Julian whistled, and he grinned at me. . . . Two days alone together, before all the summer visitors arrived.

When we reached the coast highway, I turned south, driving past ice plant and coyote bush covering the dunes, the sky a dull gray, the sea smooth and green. Wind blew through the open windows, bringing refreshing relief from the valley heat.

I parked the car in a pull-out area near Pescadero Creek, which slid hesitantly down to the sea. Stuffing two oranges and a plastic water bottle into a pack, we set out along a sandy path heading away from the ocean and skirting a marsh. Gulls flapped and screeched overhead and a snowy egret stood like a white stick against gray marsh grass.

Julian and I strolled silently hand in hand. A jumble of emotions swirled in me: happiness at hiking this trail with Julian, sadness at thinking of our life eroding away. How many more outings like this would we have?

We passed the marsh and climbed onto a rise where we looked down at a pond and the vast sea beyond. Sprawling on coarse grass, we lay together, the breeze brushing over us, delicious sun warming our skin.

"Julian," I began. "In case I never told you before . . . I've had a very privileged and comfortable life. I want to thank you."

He looked over at me and laughed.

"You sound like I'm dying or something."

"Well, I just feel enormously . . . grateful."

"It's not over, you know." Julian picked at a dried twig.

"Of course not, but it's just . . . I suddenly appreciate all I've had."

Julian snapped his twig and stared at the sea. I squirmed closer to him, lying on my back, my head resting on his belly.

"I spoiled a lot of times being angry at you," I said. "I'm sorry for the time I wasted."

He slipped his hand under my shirt.

"What I mean is, it's been good . . . you've given me so much. I feel blessed. I want to tell you . . ."

Julian rolled over to lie beside me on the grass. We lay on our backs, bodies pressed against each other, gazing up at wisps of cloud.

Later, in the motel room, we stripped off sandy clothes and stepped into a steamy shower. Pulling back the maroon flowered spread, we leapt into starched white sheets, kissed and held each other. Afterward we lay on the rumpled bed and continued our talk.

"You know," he said. "I can handle this memory thing now, as it is." He trailed his fingers through my hair. "But I'm afraid . . . it might get worse."

I lay quietly and listened. For two years I had wrestled with fears of this illness's progression while Julian never seemed to face the dreadful fact.

"But right now I'm happy," he said. "I'm a free and simple man. There's so much I want to do when I stop working."

My heart raced. "You're right, Julian. You've worked hard all your life. Now relax. Enjoy whatever you're doing. You've no pressures, no deadlines."

But he was also wrong. My hunch that he wouldn't accomplish his plans pressed on my heart. How much more time did he have?

In the motel's hot tub, we sat close to each other in steamy water on a slippery blue fiberglass ledge. Other couples talked and laughed, climbing in and out. My legs floated on the surface as I eavesdropped on their chatter, hot water absorbing my cares.

That evening at the Fish Trap, Julian and I sat across from each other over a blue cloth with a candle at the table's center. Over my broiled swordfish and his fish and chips, we talked. Cold chablis slowed us down.

We discussed things we had never talked about directly before: The certain progression of his memory problems, my anxiety over finances, the need to plan for an uncertain future. Julian listened as I shared my fears. He seemed wide open, without his usual resistance. We held hands across the table, strewn with bread crumbs, and I remembered other dinners spoiled by arguments and silly quarrels that felt so unimportant now.

Julian looked at me with clear blue eyes. "I feel so good," he said. "I'm happy. Free and healthy. I have a deep strong feeling it'll be okay."

While Julian went to the cashier to pay the bill, I put down 15 percent for the tip, a calculation I knew he could no longer make. Then we left the restaurant and stood by the black heaving sea, the night air salty, the dark sky sprinkled with stars.

He put his arm around my shoulders, and we stood together looking off into our dark anniversary night . . . the motel bed, massage oil, Baroque tapes, a book of short stories, a breakfast of lingonberries and Swedish pancakes, and tomorrow's day at the beach . . . all those many pleasures still before us.

Women Weave

The phone rang yesterday. It was Lynette, a colleague of Julian's and an old friend. She is an animal physiologist, like Julian, and directs the animal-human bond program at the University of California in Davis.

"Hi," she said. "How are you? We're just back from a six-month sabbatical in Nepal. An elephant project." Her husband, also a longtime colleague of Julian's, investigated grazing patterns of elephant herds, while Lynette interviewed elephant drivers.

As I unloaded the dryer and folded my father's laundry, she told me she was writing articles on the relationship between elephants and their owners.

"It was wonderful," she said. "I cried when I left." Then she said, "What are *you* doing? How's Julian? How are you?"

I never quite know how to answer these questions. How am I exactly? The answer changes from day to day and from hour to hour.

Shall I answer casually, "Fine"?

Shall I tell the good things that may be happening? There's always something nice: swims in the pool, walks at the Baylands, our anniversary trip. Or shall I tell her how hard some days are: the garbled conversations with Julian, the endless searching for lost objects, the ever-increasing list of things he can't do? Shall I tell her how resilient Julian is, or how exasperating? Shall I tell her how cheerful and sweet he is, or how forgetful, repetitive, simple, and confused? Shall I tell her that my father has been diagnosed with a recurrence of neck cancer? And that my sister has just returned from Ecuador and leaves in ten days for two months in Africa just before Dad's operation? Shall I tell her about the conference I'm planning for teachers on gay and lesbian youth or about how stressed and trapped I often feel?

"We're fine," I said. "Having a pleasant summer. We're chugging along."

I certainly didn't reveal how jealous I felt hearing about the elephant project. I didn't let on how humdrum my life feels, driving Julian and my father to doctor's appointments and making endless trips to grocery stores and Longs Drug.

"Are you working?" Lynette asked.

"No," I mumbled. "Not just now." In society's eyes, it seems I'm not working. I have no official job, no professional title. I get no salary, except the $18.42 royalty check I just received from my chapbook of cancer poems.

But I *am* working: to make our lives work, my own and Julian's. I design my time, creating a shape from each day's demands. My eighty-one-year-old father, with his latest health crisis looming ahead, needs me to take him to clinics. Julian needs me more and more, as he is increasingly less able to manage his life. I handle family business and attend board meetings of Parents and Friends of Lesbians and Gays. . . . Isn't this working?

"What are you doing these days?" Lynette asked me.

I felt like saying, "Maintaining." An unemployed reggae musician used to answer this question with "I'm maintaining."

Yet my life is rich. In just this week, I'm speaking to high school counselors on the lack of services for gay teenagers. I talked to distraught parents who just learned their daughter is a lesbian, set up two workshops, and planned a booth for a health fair. I answer a hotline for Parents and Friends of Lesbians and Gays and facilitate their monthly support group meeting.

I talk with Ben about graduate school. I hang out with Karen and my two grandchildren. I take my son-in-law's samba class. I have long phone conversations with Jeff in New York. I take care of myself by swimming, walking, writing, and visiting friends.

I keep the household running smoothly: cleaning, planning, arranging, repairing, organizing. I could call myself an administrator, maybe.

The summer onslaught of visitors approaches. Julian's brother and his wife come from Scotland for ten days. Jeff arrives from New York for two weeks. Ben's boyfriend from Boston will visit for a week, and Manuel and Maria from Spain will come for a month. I hope this will be fun. That's the point, after all. But houseguests require clean sheets, toilet paper, breakfasts, and dinners. My challenge is to remain peaceful, despite what exasperations each day may bring.

Yesterday, while walking in the hills behind Stanford, a friend told me what a Jungian therapist said about women's lives: that women are weavers.

Women weave life together, bit by bit, strand by strand, creating a multicolored, multitextured cloth.

Suddenly I realize what I am doing. Helping Julian and my dad, spending time with my kids, caring for Julian, and writing and doing gay advocacy work are different threads of my complex life. Each day I gather the strands presented to me at that moment and hold them in my hands, weaving them into my life's fabric.

If Lynette calls again and asks what I'm doing, I think I'll tell her, "I'm weaving."

A Moment of Laughter

I turned over onto my back and wiggled my toes. The sheets felt smooth and cool. Morning sun slanted through the window where Julian had drawn one curtain before leaving for his run. He wouldn't be back for half an hour.

Five shoes lay on the floor, one in the bookshelf and another atop the TV. Three rolled-up pairs of pants were on the chair, with two more on his dresser. Our houseguests were gone—my brother-in-law and sister-in-law back to Scotland, Manuel and Maria to the Canary Islands. Jeff was sleeping. I didn't have to be at the hospital until eleven; my dad couldn't have visitors before then. Sighing, I laced my fingers under my head and watched a black squirrel scurry along the loquat branch carrying a round yellow fruit in his mouth.

A knock on the door was followed by Jeff's voice: "Mom? You awake? Can I come in?" His footsteps padded down the hall. A spoon clinked in a cup and I smelled freshly ground coffee.

Lanky Jeff appeared at the foot of my bed wearing Julian's red striped pajamas, a perfect fit. He held a tray with two blue and white flowered mugs, a small pitcher of hot milk and the folded newspaper. "Coffee, Mom?"

"Oh, Jeff," I said. "Wow! Thank you!" I inched over and patted the bed.

He set down the tray and sat beside me, his clear blue eyes so like Julian's. But his short spiked hair stiff with gel and his gold-looped earring were distinctly Jeff. As he handed me a mug of coffee, suddenly my eyes filled with tears.

"Oh, honey," I said.

"Don't cry, Mom." Jeff looked away and busied himself stirring sugar in his cup.

"Dad brought me coffee in bed nearly every morning," I said.

Summer 1992

"I know."

"He can't make coffee anymore. He can barely put a tea bag in a cup of boiling water."

Jeff picked up the newspaper and began working the crossword. Summer session at New York's City College had just ended, and he was home for two weeks before the fall semester began. His girlfriend was handling his shifts at the Mexican restaurant where they worked.

"I'm sorry," I said. "I didn't mean to upset you."

"It's okay." His eyes focused on the *Chronicle* puzzle. "What's a four-letter word for 'cougar's bed'?"

"Don't ask me. I'm terrible at puzzles." I sipped my coffee, regretting my tears. I didn't want to overwhelm him with sadness or darken his visit with my grief. Our twenty-two-year-old, our youngest son, is the most distant from the family. Partly it's because he lives three thousand miles away, where he is deep into studying music, sound technology, computer synthesizers, and digital recording.

"New York is where I have to be," he has told me on numerous occasions.

But he also maintains an emotional distance, because he's at that stage of life when he needs to find his own way, just as Ben and Karen did at his age. They, being older, have worked through separating and are now more comfortable being close.

A pity, I've often thought, that just when I would like Jeff to recognize the limited days he has left with his dad, he needs space. I try to keep him informed without being too heavy-handed. He deserves his youth, after all. There'll be time enough to lean on him later.

Jeff continued working the puzzle. "How about six letters . . . a 'water nymph'?"

I scanned the rolled-up trousers and shoes scattered about the room. Then I noticed Julian's underpants on the bookshelf and his dresser drawers gaping open.

"Dad forgets where his clothes go. He leaves the drawers and closet open so he can see what's inside," I said, gesturing toward the chaotic scene.

Through his open closet door I saw two pairs of jeans with hangers clipping their waistbands, so that they hung down like skirts. "He's forgotten how to hang up clothes." Jeff sipped his coffee and kept working the puzzle.

"I'm sorry, Jeff. I know it upsets you to hear this. But sometimes I need to talk. And I also think you need to know."

Jeff looked up and met my eyes. "It's okay, Mom. You can talk. Do you think just because I don't write or phone much, I don't understand?"

"I know you do. . . . But you're losing your dad, at a younger age than Ben and Karen. You've had less of him. I'm sorry. . . . I wish he could talk to you about school, what you're doing, your plans. I wish he could help you."

"I've had lots of time with Dad. Maybe more than Ben or Karen."

It's true. This youngest son of ours lived alone with Julian and me the longest. His brother and sister had already left home when Jeff was in high school, leaving him with us for four years before he too went off to college. In some ways he had had more time alone with his father. Every Sunday night for years, Jeff and Julian had rolled about on our king-size bed howling with laughter over Monty Python reruns. Jeff appreciated the wry British humor that Julian loved. They knew the cheese shop, flying instructor, and Spanish Inquisition routines by heart.

"You have to accept what's happening, Mom. You can't change it." Jeff's voice deepened and took on a manly tone. "It's kind of cute the way Dad rolls up his trousers. He rolls them so neatly . . ."

The front door slammed and Julian burst into the bedroom. He peeled off his T-shirt, his bare chest glistening with sweat.

Jeff put down the crossword and held up the Datebook section. "How'd you like to go to some concerts while I'm here?" Jeff asked Julian. "The San Francisco Symphony's playing Thursday, and the Kronos Quartet's at Stanford Saturday with some Siberian 'throatsingers.' Want to go?"

As Jeff showed Julian the *Chronicle* ads I slipped out of bed, headed for the bathroom. I heard Jeff explaining as I washed and dressed.

"The concert's on Thursday, Dad. Tomorrow. Tomorrow night. We can go to the concert tomorrow night. Would you like that?"

Brushing my teeth, I thought what a "cool dude" Jeff is, with his spiked, gelled hair, his stubbly brown beard, his somewhat aloof style. On the surface, that is. Underneath is an aware, sensitive young man, not entirely comfortable talking about what's happening to Julian, but not backing off either. And accepting Julian with possibly less anguish than the rest of us.

"I'll get tickets, Dad," I heard Jeff say. Then I heard Julian giggle as Jeff launched into his version of the cheese shop skit from Monty Python.

"Well, do you have any Emmenthal, any Gorgonzola, any fontina?" Jeff said in a pompous British accent.

"Nope," said Julian.

"How about Brie, Stilton or Caerphilly?"

"Nope."

"Mozzarella?"

"Nope."

"What kind of a cheese shop is this anyway?"

And Julian and Jeff burst out laughing as I dressed and readied myself for today's trip to the hospital to visit my dad.

"Hi, Daddy"

My dad got discharged yesterday, after two weeks in the hospital for surgery on his neck cancer. When I went to get him, I found him sitting in the day room of the Extended Care Unit, dressed in his navy blue jogging suit. His white-collared polo shirt was unbuttoned, leaving an opening for the white plastic tracheotomy tube that stuck out over a clean gauze pad. His breathing was easy.

"Hi, Daddy. We're going home," I said.

He waved; it was too much trouble to cover his trach tube and speak. He motioned for me to bring him his clipboard and a pencil from his recently vacated room across the hall. The clipboard lay on his rumpled bed. The room smelled of stale urine. An elderly, gray-whiskered man lay curled on his side in the second bed, bony legs sticking out of a short blue flowered gown.

I returned to the day room and handed Dad the clipboard. "Let's get out of here," I said. "I'll bet you're glad to leave."

My dad wrote on his clipboard, "These f—— nurses don't know one end from the other!" Then he wrote, "I want out of this snake pit!"

Flipping back through the yellow lined tablet, I reread his notes to me on previous visits: "I sat in the goddamned bed for five hours and they wouldn't let me get up becuz it wasn't in the orders." "No management here. The head nurse stinks!"

My dad's been less than happy this past week in the ECU. During his first week in the hospital, he had rallied his resources: he was strong, humorous, charming. He put on his best face, my stoic father, who has gone through so much. The nurses loved him. "What a fine gentleman your dad is," they told me. "He's a really great man. We love caring for him."

And so he is. In recent years he has endured three long hospitalizations; he lay in hosital beds for months, a real trooper.

But this last week, despite steady medical progress, his spirits sank. Angry, fed up, bored, restless, uncomfortable, he let me have it whenever I came. Each day I visited, I found him "pissed as hell" about some delay or changed arrangement or ineptitude on the part of a nurse's aide.

He grew grumpier. I needed more and more patience to listen to his outbursts with understanding. I was nearly his only visitor. I'm the daughter with "discretionary time," as my cousin puts it, as she drives Los Angeles freeways for hours in different directions to help out her elderly mother, mother-in-law, and a maiden aunt.

My sister is in Africa for two months, on an expedition visiting the Rendille, a nomadic tribe in northern Kenya. She phoned from London after Dad's surgery to see how he was. Of course, she worried. When she is in town, she is caring and concerned about him and brings him weekly to her house. But for this medical round, she was gone. She left the day after his preop appointment. She told me the timing of her trip was "terrible" and she "hated leaving at a time like this." But she left.

Summer 1992

I got a postcard from Oxford, telling me how much the coun-
tryside had changed since we lived there in 1970. Then another
postcard from Kenya with a lion on it, saying she was glad the
operation had gone well and that she was leaving the next day for
the Rendille. As I read the cards, a lump formed in my throat.
What I longed to hear was that she understood and appreciated
what I was doing.

My daughter lives an hour away, juggling her busy life with
two young children, currently consumed with a martial arts festival and a group of visiting Brazilians. Jeff, who had spent eight
hours with me at the hospital the day of Dad's surgery, has
returned to New York. Ben, a major supporter, leaves soon for
Boston and is now preoccupied with his departure. Julian can't
help much. He couldn't find the hospital even if I told him where
it was, and he and my dad have little to say to each other under
the best of circumstances.

Imagine Julian, with Alzheimer's-caused aphasia, conversing
with my father, who writes notes on a clipboard and breathes
through a trach.

So it's me who visits Daddy daily, twice some days. It's me
who listens to his curses and complaints, who consoles him, com-
miserates with him, cheers him, takes him for walks, intervenes
with nurses, and talks to his doctors. After dealing daily with
Julian's confusions, the demands on my self-control run high.

Dad's discharge didn't go smoothly. One hour before he was
to leave, as he sat neatly dressed by his packed suitcase, we learned
that he couldn't return to his retirement home with a trach. State
regulations require that retirement homes cannot house people with
tracheotomies, even if they're temporary. I was furious, flooded by
the terrible feeling that he might end up coming home with me.

"No! No!" I cried to the discharge planner, the retirement
home manager, and the head nurse. "My husband has Alzheimer's.
I can't take care of my husband *and* my father. Soon you'd have to
look for a placement for me!"

A flurry of phone calls finally achieved permission for him to
return to his retirement home, on "borrowed time." He could be
put out any day.

But home we went to his bright, sunny apartment that he loves, my mother's vases and his second wife's carved Chinese figures prominently displayed. Pictures of Julian and me, my sister and her husband, grandchildren and great-grandchildren, adorn the refrigerator door. Framed photos of his three wives sit on his dresser. Of course he wanted to go home.

After spending the afternoon helping a visiting nurse settle him into his apartment, I escaped to Stanford for a swim and a quick nap on the grass by the pool. Then I returned to help Dad get ready for bed. That's when the night ordeal started.

My father really can't care for his trach, supposedly a requirement before going home. I don't know how to care for it either. What is this suction machine that looms by his bed, the long plastic tubes and blue hoses, the boxes of sterilized suction equipment? How do I operate the mist machine that is supposed to provide him cool, moist air at night through his trach to prevent his secretions from drying out, clogging his tube and choking him?

No one showed me how to operate all this paraphernalia, as they were supposed to do, I learned later. I'm no good with physical crises and medical equipment.

As I helped Dad undress, new duties began: slip off his shirt without dislodging the trach, ask him to wipe his secretions, tighten the neck strap holding the plastic tube in place. Each act made him cough and wheeze.

When I finally placed the mist mask over his trach, it didn't fit. The clasp was broken and the mask wouldn't stay in place. The respiratory therapist hadn't called as the visiting nurse said he would. Mist wasn't coming through the blue plastic tube.

"Oh shit!" my father said.

Exhaling slowly, I settled my dad, brought more pillows, and tried again to attach the mist machine while staring at the ominous-looking suction equipment by the bed. Julian, who had returned with me "just to say good night," could do nothing to help.

"You said we'd only be here twenty minutes," Julian complained from the couch where he lay watching TV.

It was eleven P.M. I phoned the equipment rental agency and spoke to two operators and a dispatcher, who finally put me in touch with the respiratory therapist who had delivered the equipment. He talked me through how to repair the broken clasp and adjust the mist meter. I felt as if I were in an airplane, the pilot had collapsed, and the control tower was instructing me over a radio how to land.

I hate this, I muttered to myself. I don't like equipment! I never wanted to be a nurse! I'm scared for Daddy. What if he chokes in the night? Someone should sleep here. That someone could only be me. But I don't want to sleep here. I'm afraid. Where is everybody?

"Come on, let's go," Julian called from the sofa. I felt torn. Part of me felt I needed to sleep in my dad's apartment on his sofa bed, where I could listen to his breathing, hear if he is getting enough air, know if he is strangling. I should stay and help him suction himself if he needs to, but I don't know how. He can't really do it either. I wanted to go to my own house and sleep in my own bed, where I wouldn't have to listen to his strident, labored breathing and his violent coughing, gagging attacks. I felt afraid to go and afraid to stay.

My father finally maneuvered himself into bed. He breathed easily. The mist machine hummed, the clasp held, the blue plastic tube leading from the machine to the opening in his neck grew cloudy. The gauge pointed to the exact number the respiratory therapist had told me on the phone. I remembered that the ECU nurses said he had had no trouble breathing the past four nights. He had slept straight through and hadn't needed suctioning. I consoled myself. He had only to push the bell and someone from the night desk would come to his room and they could call me or 9-1-1.

I imagined my bed at home with its flowered spread and comforting pillows. I longed to be alone. I longed to rest. I decided to leave. I kissed my dad's whiskered cheek. He breathed easily and looked relaxed.

"Goodnight, Daddy. You're looking great," I said. "Sure you feel okay? Would you like me to stay?"

He shook his head and gave me his thumbs-up sign. I switched on the kitchen light and went back one more time to check the mist machine. Conflicted as I was, I walked out the door toward the elevator, Julian behind me.

"Push 'Lobby,'" I said.

Downstairs, cool night air washed over me as Julian and I left the retirement complex and headed for the car. The black sky glittered with stars.

"You said we'd only be there fifteen minutes," Julian said. "We were there two hours!"

At home I slept fitfully. Maybe I should have stayed with my father? Next morning, as soon as I woke up, I phoned him.

"Daddy, hi. How are you?" I made my voice casual to camouflage how anxious I felt.

Relief flooded me as I heard his voice, fairly clear, not so gurgly, reassuringly familiar.

"I'm okay. Had a good night. Thank you, darling," my father said.

Visiting the Hyenas

The first hyena lay on her side in the straw just near the fence of the enclosure. She raised her head when we stopped in front of her. Her pup crawled out from under her back leg where he had been nursing, black and cuddly looking, his fur fluffy and his eyes round and black. They both stared at me with huge, dark eyes.

"Don't put your hands on the fence," Laurence Frank warned. He confessed that his own six-year-old daughter had had the tip of her third finger bitten off recently. She had been watching a hyena and innocently grasping the cyclone fence as she looked.

Laurence Frank runs the hyena project at the University of California in Berkeley, where thirty hyenas live in a field station high in the Berkeley hills. Julian and I had spent three weeks camping with Laurence in Kenya ten years ago, observing hyenas in the flat grasslands of the Masai-Mara game preserve near the Serengeti.

Last Sunday, Laurence invited Julian and me to see the hyenas and spend the day with him and the psychology professor, Steve Glickman, who heads the project. A dear friend of Julian's,

Irv Zucker, had invited us all to dinner afterward. I sensed that they had created this day as a gift to Julian.

As we drove to Berkeley, I repeated the names of the men we would see: Laurence, Steve, Irv. Julian wrote the names on a scrap of paper and studied them.

"Laurence?" He looked at me quizzically as I drove across the Bay Bridge. "Who's Laurence?"

"You remember when we went to Kenya with Laurence Frank," I said. "Remember we camped with Laurence on the game preserve and studied hyenas?" I was shocked that he couldn't connect the name Laurence with our great adventure, which he was also struggling to recall.

Once Laurence walked down the path in his Levis, denim shirt, and Birkenstocks, greeted us at the main gate and embraced us, Julian remembered.

Julian and I strolled through the field station with Laurence and Steve. In the first cage a black newborn pup crawled out from under her tawny, spotted mother. Next to her another female lay with two-week-old twins.

Then we saw a pair of young males, Masai and Mara. As we passed their enclosure they bounded over to the fence, reared up on hind legs, and nuzzled the gate, their hay-colored fur the same color as the dried grass in the enclosure. Their huge jaws opened, showing powerful teeth, capable of chewing and grinding the bones of a zebra or antelope. Calcium-rich white scat, almost pure chalk from the bones they crunch and eat, lay on the ground. When Laurence lectures on the hyena's digestive system, he writes on the blackboard and later explains that the chalk he is using is hyena shit.

Laurence told anecdotes about each hyena, describing its personality and pausing to pet and fondle each one as we passed its enclosure. He has hand-fed many of them since infancy, with a bottle. Only Laurence enters the cages of these animals others fear to touch. Everyone, including Laurence, has been bitten.

Laurence Frank is a field biologist who lived for years in Kenya, camping on the savannah, studying the social behavior of a hyena clan. He and Julian met at a conference on the behavioral effects of testosterone, Julian's area of expertise, and Laurence consulted Julian on how androgens affect sexual behavior.

Hyenas are strange creatures. Males and females look alike, but unlike most mammals, female hyenas are larger than the males, more aggressive and dominant. They have an amazing "pseudo-phallus" and a scrotum, an empty sack that hangs between their hind legs. In social-greeting rituals, females actually get erections. The pseudo-phallus is, mysteriously, the vagina, and pups are born through it.

So in 1982 Laurence invited Julian to the Masai-Mara. The plan was to shoot females with tranquilizers, anesthetize them, and take blood samples, which Julian would carry back to Stanford. Then Julian's lab would analyze the hormone levels to see if high testosterone in the blood of female hyenas might explain their large size and dominant, aggressive behavior over males.

Of course, I insisted on going! While I rarely accompanied Julian to professional meetings, I was not going to miss camping in Africa with Laurence and observing hyenas. Those three weeks turned out to be the most exciting of my life, and for Julian a scientific adventure outside his less exotic research with rats in Stanford labs.

Now, ten years later, the hyena research continues in the Berkeley hills. A large research program developed from Laurence and Julian's project. Eventually Julian introduced Laurence to Steve, head of the University of California psychology department, and together they wrote grants and got funding, built the field station, and brought baby hyenas from Kenya to Berkeley.

Strolling through the field station, Laurence and Steve talked to Julian about the project. I asked a lot of questions while Julian walked along fairly quiet. Laurence and Steve talked enthusiastically. They looked at Julian and spoke directly to him, telling him this or that, but I saw that he barely understood what they were saying.

They were great with him, aware, of course, of his language problems, but it wasn't the same. Julian couldn't discuss androgen receptors or the neurochemistry of testosterone. He listened, smiled, made a remark or two, a general, vague statement to camouflage his uncertainty. But their conversation was a simple, superficial parody of the excited scientific debates they used to have, when ideas flew back and forth, references to recent papers were cited, and suggestions were made for future projects.

The visit bothered me more than it did Julian. His eyes lit up. He mumbled about doing something with the hyena project during these last months before he retires. He is worried about what he'll do after his sabbatical officially ends this August until his lab shuts down in April. It's eight months, after all, and Julian has never been idle.

"Maybe our lab can get involved in some way," Julian said, his eyes bright with enthusiasm, the old light on again about science.

"You're welcome anytime," Laurence and Steve said.

After we toured the animal compound, they took us to the operating room and labs. They showed us a film of the birth of a pup: the black, slimy, wet newborn hyena slipping out through its mother's erect phallus/vagina. Steve and Laurence narrated this amazing video, telling us story after story about hyenas in the wild.

Pangs of sadness and yearning washed over me; if Julian felt sad, it didn't show. But I felt his loss. He is no longer one of the bright, competent scientists. He is too young to be so out of it, yet that's not the point. When he retired, he should have been able to remain active. Instead, all his knowledge is gone. Still, I remind myself, he is respected for the work he has done and what he has contributed. I tell him this often. He has had a productive, creative career. It's okay to stop.

After the hyena visit, the four of us drove to Irv's house high in the Berkeley hills. Irv had engineered this excursion, I realized, and invited everyone back to his house for dinner. The three wives joined us for drinks on Irv's deck, which extends out over a steep slope. The bay, the bridge, and the skyline of San Francisco spread out before us, golden in the setting sun.

Chilled chardonnay. Sesame crackers and Brie. Salmon dip and jicama and guacamole. And talk. The easy, bright banter of clever people: what's happening with the hyenas, how the renewal of funding is going, how Ross Perot's withdrawal from the presidential race will affect the election.

Julian sat quietly, sipping his wine. He couldn't keep up with the quick exchange. He couldn't formulate his thoughts fast enough to enter this conversation. He couldn't grasp the essence of the discussion. He couldn't find the right words. So he remained silent. I chattered on, contributing for both of us, including him whenever I could:

"Julian did this or that . . . ," I said. "Julian feels . . . Julian says . . ." or "Remember when . . ." I rescued Julian when he did attempt a sentence or two or when he stumbled over a word. It wasn't relaxing. I felt tense and sad. No longer were we a competent couple like these other bright couples. No more dinner parties for us, evenings with people discussing interesting things. We mostly walk, watch videos, go to concerts, hike or bike ride, where intellectual and verbal demands are less.

Our friends were kind. They included Julian. They spoke directly to him and responded to his statements with interest even when his remarks were off the subject.

The talk turned to a well-known animal behaviorist in their department who died several years ago, the grandfather of their field. They discussed how hard it was for him when he retired. Even though he remained wise and knowledgeable, fully competent, writing and working until his final illness, the spark went out.

"His self-esteem plummeted after he retired," Irv said.

"It was hard to let go," I said. "But it's part of life. The challenge is to let go with pride and find new things to do." It occurred to me that each person around that table was terrified over what was happening to Julian. It was hard for those dominant males, those testosterone-laden, competitive, accomplished men to imagine being less than what they were.

"I'm proud of Julian," I said. "He is learning to let go and feel happy with new activities." I worried that Julian might be embarrassed over my exposing him, but he continued drinking his wine and spreading guacamole on crackers.

Then I told them about Thich Nhat Hanh. I attempted to imitate his Vietnamese accent, saying: "It's in our nature to grow old. It's in our nature to have ill health. In our nature to watch our loved ones change and leave us. In our nature to die," I said. "Julian and I are practicing letting go and enjoying life in new ways."

I'm not sure why I interjected this into the conversation. I think I wanted to validate Julian and our present life.

Everyone stared at me as I spoke. They didn't say anything. I didn't know what they were feeling. Did they think I was preachy, inappropriate, or a Pollyanna? Never mind. This was what Julian and I were doing. Why shouldn't I talk about it?

I recalled Laurence in the Mara, driving his Land Rover over the grasslands, one hand on the steering wheel, the other holding binoculars, tracking hyenas across the savannah. I imagined Steve, lecturing at Berkeley and managing the field station. I thought of Irv and his teaching, his research, his competence, and his bright, funny repartee. Then I thought of Julian singing in the Yiddish Chorus and handing out sugar and eggs at the Food Closet, where he volunteers. Now he can hardly make a pot of coffee.

But in an odd way, we are still happy. If I don't focus on all that we've lost, if I don't compare his life now to what it was, if I stay truly present and tune in to the small, daily joys that are always here, then I'm okay. For some strange reason, we are actually happier at times than we were when we operated at our peak, now that everything is precarious and threatened, now that I'm so aware of impermanence.

In the car driving home, Julian said, "I need to be useful. I also need excitement." He has had both in his long career. The Food Closet now satisfies his need to be useful, but it's certainly not exciting.

Maybe we could visit the hyenas occasionally. Maybe Julian could accept Laurence's offer to hang around the field station. Only he would have to remember to keep his fingers outside the cyclone fence.

How Far I've Come

Yesterday I went to the Veteran's Hospital to hear Nancy Mace, author of *The Thirty-Six-Hour Day: A Family Guide for Caring for People With Alzheimer's.*

"This book is the caregivers' bible," said the psychiatric nurse who introduced her before the lecture.

Alzheimer's, A Love Story

Sitting in the audience, I realized that two years ago, when Julian was first diagnosed, I was so horrified, I couldn't read that book. I forced myself to read only the chapters on financial and legal planning.

I used to look at Julian's sleeping face next to mine on the pillow, remember the Alzheimer's Association pamphlets, and shudder. I imagined him mute, vacant, incontinent, not knowing me, feeling a horror beyond anything I'd ever known.

One year later, I finally dared to read *The Thirty-Six-Hour Day*, in 1991, during a week I spent alone in the mountains at Kit Carson. I read it and wept. But it made perfect sense. By then I had accepted that this was to be our life, in some form or other. A year earlier I could only wail: "No! Not Julian! Not me!" Now, here I was ready to hear Nancy Mace, author of that book, talk to caregivers.

As she spoke Nancy Mace held up a model of a human brain enclosed in a plastic skull. She removed the frontal lobes and the convoluted cortex and showed us the visual cortex and parietal lobes. She pointed to parts of the brain where different functions were controlled.

"Think of a couple watching television one evening," she said. "They get hungry and decide to make a roast beef sandwich during the commercial. They go to the kitchen and get out the necessary items: bread, mayonnaise, lettuce, tomato, meat, knife, plate. They make the sandwich, return to the living room, watch the end of the program, and clean the kitchen after the show ends.

"Simple enough. We do things like this every day," she said. Then she explained step-by-step what happens to cognitively impaired people. She explained why dementia patients break down and why they do the odd things that they do.

"People with dementia have trouble planning, postponing, anticipating and choosing," Nancy Mace said. She explained why Alzheimer's patients can't choose or select from an array of choices: clothes in the closet, food on a menu. "They can't make decisions, can't regulate or order their thoughts. They can't sequence events properly. They do things in the wrong order. They can't start activities and can't stop."

As Nancy Mace kept using the word "can't," I thought how for Julian, it's not yet "can't." This disease is a process, a matter of degree. I know we're on a downhill slide. But where we are now, it's more accurate to say "has trouble with." "Julian has trouble with . . . ," I often tell friends who ask how he is. Julian has trouble handling money, making coffee, putting gas in the car.

"People with Alzheimer's have agnosias," Nancy Mace continued. They fail to comprehend the meaning of objects, faces, and words. That's why Alzheimer's patients forget how to use familiar tools. They don't know what to do with a fork or razor. They may say to their wife of forty years, "Who are you? Why are you getting into my bed?" A spoken word suddenly loses its meaning as if it's gibberish or Chinese.

"People with dementia can't select or filter what's significant from the huge array of events happening around us all the time," she said. "They can't ignore the irrelevant and focus on the relevant."

Nancy Mace spoke of quick feelings of irritation. She said, "Their brain lies to them." They don't grasp the significance of situations. Their feedback systems have failed. Impulse control is lost. They are unable to repress or hold back irritation. She kept reminding us, "They can't help this. There's organic, structural loss to the brain."

A man raised his hand and asked the origin of the word "Alzheimer's."

"Alzheimer's disease was first described by a German physician, Alois Alzheimer, in 1907," she said. "And the condition was named for him." She explained that he had examined a woman in her early fifties and called her condition "presenile dementia." But neurologists now call it "senile dementia of the Alzheimer's type," both in younger and elderly patients.

The conference room at the VA was packed, nearly every chair taken. As Nancy Mace spoke, a tanned, gray-haired man and his wife entered the room. She shuffled in with the familiar stoop I now recognize. Her hair was short, straight, unbrushed. She looked unkempt, as if he were dressing her and doing her hair. He led her toward two empty chairs near me and pointed.

"Sit down," he said. "Sit down."

"Damn. Damn it to hell," she muttered. "I want to go home." The man shushed her, leaned over, and whispered in her ear. She said loudly, "I want to go home."

Nancy Mace, right in the middle of a sentence, smiled at the man and said, "We're glad to have you. We don't mind a bit that she is talking. It won't bother us. We're glad she's here."

The man's face softened. He looked relieved. I felt glad I hadn't brought Julian.

"Long-term memory is better for a while," Nancy Mace continued. "But eventually they lose this too.

"The internal clock breaks down," she said. "They lose their sense of time. They repeat questions endlessly, unaware that time has passed.

"These functions are lost unevenly," she said. "Many patients may have good social skills. Doctors, visiting relatives, and friends are often fooled. The person may be charming and behave pretty well in limited social settings. You need to be around for a while to really understand."

Looking around the audience, I saw several spouses from the couples group, but I was surprised to see patients too. When the talk ended, I asked one woman why she had brought her husband.

"Isn't it depressing for him to hear this?"

"Oh, he doesn't understand the lecture," she said. "He just likes to be in the crowd."

But Julian isn't at this stage yet, I thought. He would understand all too well. Seeing the disheveled woman act strangely would upset him. So would Nancy Mace's words. He is struggling hard to hang on to his normal life.

Each person with Alzheimer's is somewhere on the bumpy road from normalcy to oblivion. Each person in this room came because they themselves or someone they love is on this downhill slide.

"Managing emotions is one of the hardest tasks," Nancy Mace continued. "If either the patient or the caregiver isn't angry," she said, "then one of you is depressed.

"You are all courageous," she went on, looking from face to face in the audience.

Yes, yes, I thought. I feel toward this audience as I feel toward folks in other support groups I've been in: Parents and Friends of Lesbians and Gays and my previous breast cancer group. Members of any support group are on a common journey, even though each person is in a different place. It's comforting to be together with others who understand.

Only with Alzheimer's, there's no hope of things improving. There's only certain decline and the awesome, continual task of acceptance. It's frightening to look ahead. In the couples' group I've watched the frazzled, sad, frantic, panicky, exhausted expressions in caregivers' faces. I wonder how I'll cope?

Frightening as it is, coming to lectures links me to others on this Alzheimer's path. As Nancy Mace said, we *are* courageous. Yet I see joyfulness and humor, too. I marvel at the caregivers' resilience, their creativity in managing ever-changing problems. From them, I gather humanity and a little strength.

Two years ago I couldn't open Nancy Mace's book. One year ago I read it and cried. Now here I was listening to her speak, nodding my head vigorously after every sentence. I belonged in this audience of caregivers and I felt inspired to do my best. How far I've come. How far I've yet to go.

Happily Dancing the Samba

Walking into Studio J toward Beiçola's samba class, we heard the drum, its beat insisting that my body move. Opening the door, I saw the studio filled with dancers, mostly women in black tights and leotards with colorful bandanas tied around their waists. Sweat dampened their faces and darkened their shirts.

My son-in-law Beiçola (pronounced Bay-*so*-la) faced the class of twenty dancers, his back to a mirror that ran along the front wall. In loose red cotton pants and a black tank top, he swung his hips from side to side, now forward and back. All eyes were on him. He changed the step; everyone followed. He established a pattern and the class copied each new rhythm. One-two-three-sweep. One-two-three-sweep.

Beiçola waved at Julian, Ben, and me and grinned, his big

smile covering half his face, his body never breaking the beat. We inched through the door and sat quietly on the floor against the back wall. My daughter, Karen, left her spot in the first row and bounded over to greet us, her slim legs in purple tights, beads of perspiration dripping down her bare arms and shoulders above her red sleeveless leotard. Her waist-long brown hair was pulled back into a thick braid that swung from side to side as she ran.

We took off our shoes and leaned against the wall to watch. We had intended to get here by eleven so that Ben could take the class. But traffic on the freeway and an accident on the Bay Bridge made us late.

"I won't go into a dance class late," Ben told us on the drive to Berkeley. "You need to warm up properly. You need to stretch."

Ben had danced in New York for three years; he'd taken dance workshops and performed. I respected his opinion, but I also knew Beiçola. He gets everyone to dance. I suspected that Beiçola would never let Ben just sit and watch.

Sure enough. No sooner did we sit down than Beiçola sambaed his way through three lines of side-stepping, hip-swinging students to where we sat. He took Ben's hand and pulled him up. Ben protested feebly but Beiçola exaggerated his steps and pulled Ben into the line.

But then Beiçola pulled me up too. I felt only one pang of self-conscious shyness. One second of those old crippling voices: "You can't dance. You're too fat. You'll look silly. You're too old. Everyone else is slim and sexy. Look how they swing their hips. You can't do that!"

In the past those voices crippled me. They kept me sitting on sidelines bathed in negative thoughts when my body, I see now, longed to be free.

So I got up and stood in the back row watching the feet of the woman before me, trying to copy what she did.

Beiçola pulled Julian up too, conspicuous in his faded jeans, orange T-shirt, and navy socks. Everyone else was barefoot. Julian and I were twenty years older than anyone in the class.

Beiçola returned to the front of the room, laughing, grinning, changing the steps. "One-two-three-four. One-two-three-four," he sang. He sambaed into the ranks to place his hands on one woman's hips which were angled sideways, and gently repositioned them to face forward.

Julian was smiling, dancing in happy abandon. His body hung loose and floppy, his arms swinging, his feet shifting weight. He moved to the rhythm. Not exactly samba, for sure, but he was into it, bouncing to the beat.

He threw back his head, closed his eyes, and danced, looking like an older, gray-haired, gray-bearded version of his hippie self in the sixties. He danced the way he had back in those days when he loved to smoke a little pot and dance away at parties, while I remained frozen in self-critical paralysis on the sidelines, usually standing by the food table, busying myself with another turkey sandwich, more corn chips and guacamole, another brownie. Hopefully in a deep conversation, but never dancing.

While Julian closed his eyes and stomped away, I concentrated on following the steps. Right step forward, left step back, right forward, left back. Reverse. Julian swung his arms and stamped his feet, looking a little like the scarecrow in the *The Wizard of Oz*. I watched Beiçola's feet, trying to make mine do what his did. I watched his strong legs in constant motion, his muscles tighten in his red pants, his powerful lean hips.

Then he changed the pace and led the class in new steps across the floor, establishing ever-changing patterns. The class formed four lines behind him. Across the room we went. I stared at Beiçola, willing my body to look like his. Far from it.

Beiçola: tall, muscular, powerful, dark, moving rhythmically, effortlessly, energetically, smoothly, his feet accomplishing quicker and more intricate steps. Me: short, overweight, out of shape, slow, doing only a vague approximation of Beiçola's movements.

As I danced toward my reflection in the mirror, I saw a smiling, laughing woman, awkward and stiff, but moving. No samba, maybe, but I was dancing.

Beiçola came to Julian and me, exaggerating his steps so that we could follow. Ben danced well; he imitated Beiçola's movements quickly. He managed his hips, his arms looked right. I loved watching him. I watched Karen too. Her long purple legs did the steps a little slower than Beiçola, clearly comfortable with these rhythms. I scanned the samba students, picking out ones whose movements I could follow. I was sweating now, my T-shirt dark with perspiration, my hair wet, my neck dripping.

Beiçola changed the record, introducing new rhythms. Sometimes he had us pair off in couples. I danced with Julian, with Karen, and with Beiçola, moving, stepping, sliding, turning, dipping, sweeping forward, sweeping back. I felt wordlessly free and happy. Julian, too, looked carefree and well.

The routines grew faster and more intricate. Julian and I hung behind as the class continued to cross the room in even more complicated steps. Deep knee bends now. Knees touching the floor briefly, then quickly back up. We stood by the electric fan in the corner, letting the wind cool our hot faces and sweaty necks.

"If the samba class were closer to Stanford," I told Julian, "I'd come every week."

Julian nodded. "The main thing now is to have fun," he said.

There I was in Beiçola's class—with my son, my daughter, my new Brazilian son-in-law, and my husband—dancing samba. What strange behavior for descendants of dutiful, book-bound European Jews. And why not? We've been serious and heady far too long.

To paraphrase Ray Bolger, the Scarecrow in the *The Wizard of Oz*, who sang, "I could dance away the hours, looking at the flowers . . . if I only had a brain." He was wrong. It's having less brain that lets us enjoy the flowers and get into the dance.

"I Love You, Julian"

Morning sun slants through the loquat tree outside my window. Light falls in lines on the rust carpet of my bedroom and on my oak dresser drawers. I snuggle deeper into my pillow. It's Friday, my first free day in a long time. No visitors. No appointments. No phone calls. No urgent needs of my sick father's. I can shape the day however I please.

Julian appears by the bedside holding two coffee mugs. He hasn't brought me coffee for months. I'm in a half daze, that early morning twilight zone, not quite awake and not asleep.

Summer 1992

Julian sits on his side of the bed, drinking coffee and munching toast. He holds some papers in his hand.

"You know that thing where you eat and then they give you to go from one place to another." He points to the papers. Because I don't have my glasses on, I can't read, so I let him continue.

"You . . . you eat . . . and then you . . . walk. You eat and you eat and then you want to walk somewhere and you can walk somewhere because they give it to you because you ate."

I just lie there, sip my coffee, and listen. I think I'm being patient because I'm lying still and letting him say what he is trying to say. I don't interrupt, shout, or snap at him. But I know I closed my eyes twice and sighed as he floundered for a word, a word which made no sense even when he finally produced it.

"That thing—you know that thing where you don't pay but you do pay and then when you want to walk somewhere you can because you ate. . . ."

My body tightens. My mouth gets pinched. I squeeze my eyes shut. With all the summer visitors in the house these past weeks, I was rarely alone with Julian. I usually jumped up early to water the garden, lay out breakfast, make necessary phone calls, and arrange the day. The houseguests talked with Julian or we spoke in groups. Julian and I were hardly alone together, and we had no time to handle affairs or discuss our business.

As he struggles to express himself, I realize that during these busy weeks, I hadn't felt the strain of being unable to communicate with Julian. Many others were here to talk with him. The price of having visitors is no time alone. But the price of being alone is once again facing the changes in Julian. With the commotion of kids, houseguests, and my dad's operation, I had almost forgotten.

Through my blurry vision, I notice the blue and gold Visa card logo in the corner of the paper he holds. "You mean the Visa card?" I take a wild guess. "Are you talking about the Visa card where you get frequent flyer miles?"

"Frequent flyer?" He looks at me quizzically.

"Some Visa cards give you free mileage on airlines for each dollar you spend. Is that what you mean?" I ask somewhat sharply.

[71]

He throws the papers down on the bed. "Here, you read it," he says.

But I don't want to read the papers. Julian used to track the frequent flyer accounts. Often when I feel tense, impatient, or exasperated, I realize I'm bumping once again into an area he used to handle. I'm pushed to face those parts of our life where I've been dependent.

Julian finishes his coffee and leaves the room. He doesn't kiss me or say his usual "Bye, see you at suppertime, have a nice day."

When I get out of bed, he is gone. I know I've hurt him. He has slunk away.

My closest family—Julian and my father—are men I can't talk to. Julian, with his garbled, convoluted, simple efforts. My dad, with his terse, curt, irritable, snappy remarks, often curses. Neither can I talk easily with my only sister. No wonder my phone bill to my daughter across the bay is so large. We talk almost daily, I realize, often at expensive times. I chat with her on my portable phone while I make dinner, empty the dishwasher, or rest on the couch. Sometimes we talk in bed late at night, telling each other the news of our days.

I feel sad hurting Julian. Beneath irritation lies my loneliness in thinking of the friend I have lost. But I would rather feel sad and lonely than have only anger erupt. My dad expresses mainly anger, no matter what emotion he feels: confusion, uncertainty, fear, loneliness, discouragement, sadness. Mostly anger comes out.

Lying in bed, watching dust motes dance on sunbeams streaming in through my window, I dial Julian's office. I want to say I'm sorry. I don't like these spats. No one answers.

Around nine, as I'm making the bed, the phone rings. Julian's voice is soft. In a low tone, he says, "Hi. How are you? Why do you shout at me like that? I can't help it. Is it so terrible that I talk slow?"

"I didn't shout, Julian." I begin to cry. "I'm sorry I hurt your feelings. I know you're sensitive. It's just so sad. I'm sad for you . . . for me and for what's happening to our life." As I speak I think of friends our age full of plans and projects, competent, intelligent, capable people.

"Is it so bad how I talk?"

"It's not just talking," I try to explain. "It's other changes too."
Now, why did I say that? Immediately I chastise myself. What's
the point of telling him about his limitations? Part of me wants to
warn him, I guess, so that he'll be more cautious and won't drive
off alone to Berkeley or San Francisco. Or buy a ticket to "somewhere exciting," as he often threatens to do.

"I love you, Julian," I say into the phone. "I'm sad about
what's happening."

"I love you, too." His voice is tender and sweet. I know he
means it. I begin to cry. Tears roll down my cheeks and splash
onto the phone. "I love you, Julian."

"Let's not be sad," he says. "I know. I understand it all. But
let's be happy in the rest of our life."

Fall 1992

It's the turning time.

"You Should Write About It, Man"

We sprawled on the grass in Mark's garden under the apple tree, Julian, Mark, and me. Our faces soaked up warm September sun, our eyes gazed out at the deep blue cove dotted with sailboats and at the steep, wooded mountains beyond.

Mark leaned on one elbow and shoved a few marijuana leaves into his pipe. The long tapered leaves were still green. He had just pulled up the plant the day before and hung it in his shed to dry. In order to smoke these, he had put them in the microwave for three minutes.

Mark lit the pipe, inhaled deeply, and passed the pipe to me. I inhaled gently, once, just enough to accept his offering and maybe enough to enjoy a slight high. I haven't smoked for years, really. The last few times I mostly fell asleep. Julian took several puffs and lay back down, a wide grin on his face. He looked happy and relaxed. Carefree. And why not? We are visiting our old, ex-hippie friend Mark, who now lives on a small wooded island west of Vancouver.

"Tell me what it's like, man," Mark said to Julian. "Tell me what it's like when you can't find a word. Tell me. Tell me. So I can know." Mark sat up and moved close to Julian, who lay sprawled on his back, face to the sun.

"I love you, Julian," Mark said. "I want to know. I want to know what it feels like to be you."

"The words just disappear," Julian said. "I have an idea. I start to say something. And the words fly away. While I'm thinking of the word, the thought goes too."

"Tell me more, Julian. What else? Tell me." Mark sat cross-legged close to Julian, looking intently at his face. I lay quietly, trying to leave this conversation to them.

Julian spoke about how hard it is for him to talk, especially in groups. He lay on the grass, now so relaxed that he often just laughed in response to Mark's earnest questions.

"It's fucking interesting, man," Mark said. "I want to know what it's like to be you."

My chest filled with nameless emotion. Mark cared and he wasn't afraid. Not afraid to ask and not afraid to hear the answer.

"The way I see it, " Mark said, "you're still you. So you used to be a full professor at Stanford. You were the smartest one of us all. Now you can't talk well anymore. But you're still you."

Tears welled up in my eyes at hearing Mark say what I so often feel. Here was Mark, an old friend who had lived in Palo Alto in the early seventies, in those crazy days of marijuana and occasional LSD, experimenting with whatever new substances and human growth experiences happened by. Here was Mark, whom we'd hardly seen in ten years and who only learned about Julian's diagnosis two hours before we got on the ferry to visit him, here on this island where he lives with his wife, Valerie, and two small sons. Here was Mark, knowing about Julian's Alzheimer's for only a few hours, and he was "getting it."

As Julian sank into a hazy, drowsy reverie, I spoke for him. I told Mark how Julian was afraid of silence, how terrified he was of becoming mute, how frightened he was at the thought of being unable to communicate.

"There are three possibilities," Mark said. "One. That you'll have your normal keen intelligence trapped in a paralyzed body, unable to speak. Two. That when you reach the stage where you can't talk, you won't know or care about it either. Three. You die."

Pow. He just said it. Mark articulated bluntly these thoughts that had loomed black and unmentionable in both Julian's and my minds for months, maybe a year. He jumped right into our fears. He was talking, after half a day's visit, of things we'd spent months cautiously approaching and only recently putting into words.

"As far as I know, number one won't happen. That isn't Alzheimer's. You won't have your normal intelligence and sense of yourself and be unable to speak. That would be torture. But that isn't it."

I sat up, took off my sandals and felt the warm grass soft under my feet.

"Number three. You die. Well, we all die. So number two is what you face. If and when you can't talk, you won't care about it either."

Terrifying to hear him say this. Yet comforting too. Terrifying to walk up to the edge of the abyss and peer right in. Comforting to have a friend dare to walk up and peer in with us.

I inched closer to Mark. Julian lay on his back, his eyes closed, face toward the light, like a sunflower. I sat close to Mark and put my hand on his shoulder.

"Mark," I said. I wanted to tell him something. I wasn't sure what. Emotion choked off the words. Tears trickled down my cheeks.

"Cry later," Mark said. "Tell me. Give me information. Speak."

I told him we are trying to learn how to be silent without fear. We want to learn about silence. And love. We're trying to replace fearful images of being mute with positive ones of a meditating Buddha. We joke about Julian going into a cave and sitting cross-legged in silence. And me bringing him food. But it's serious, too.

"Mark," I sniffled. "Thank you. Thank you for not being afraid. Thank you for making yourself open to this pain. Most people are afraid to come too close or hear too much. It's lonely when you feel others don't understand."

I could hardly get the words out.

"Julian's so sweet," Mark said. "He's changed and not changed. What's gone is his biting intellect, his sarcasm, his skeptical, questioning response to things people say. He's dropped his fierce edge. All his gentleness shows."

I wept hearing Mark say what I know is true.

"What I see," Mark continued, "is that he searches for words. He can't express himself clearly, he can't understand everything and he gets confused. But he's really still there."

Sometimes Mark said "he" and looked at me. Sometimes he said "you" and looked at Julian. The conversation was shifting from Julian to me, partly because Julian was sleepy and stoned and had retreated into a drowsy, sun-drenched stupor on the grass. Partly because Julian was probably embarrassed at revealing himself and discussing his problems.

I wanted Julian to stay in the conversation. Julian and I talk often about these things. But rarely do we share it with others. Here was Mark, right into it with us.

"You should write about it, man," Mark said. "Write about what you think and feel. Tell us your perceptions, man. You're fucking interesting. It might be the best writing you've ever done. Fuck the hundred and seventy scientific papers on the sex life of a rat. Write about what it's like to be you!"

"He is," I said. "He's trying to write, only it's hard." I told him about Julian's autobiography project. I told him it's getting harder for Julian to write. How we're now taping interviews and transcribing them. How I think telling his story might also help others.

Mark's wife, Valerie, walked across the lawn in black tights and a blue sweater. Their two little blond boys dashed about the garden naked except for the Batman capes streaming behind them.

"I've put the chicken in the oven. We'll eat soon," Valerie said, turning back toward the house.

Mark, Julian, and I sat in a circle on the lawn, cross-legged, our knees touching. Part of me felt I should get up and help Valerie in the kitchen. I remembered too well those years when Julian and Mark would smoke dope and carry on crazy, intense, intellectual conversations while I prepared meals and wrestled my three children into pajamas.

"I should go help Valerie," I said, "but I want to stay here." I didn't want to let go of these moments.

I wanted to tell Mark some things he didn't see. I wanted to tell him how Julian can't drive, how he gets lost, how he can't read a map, how he can't handle money, how he has trouble telling time, how nine times out of ten he doesn't remember his own address. I wanted to tell him Julian can't solve simple problems, can't make or remember a plan. I wanted to tell him I had had to write "Mark and Valerie" on a page in his notebook before we came so that he could remember whom we were going to see. It took Julian hours to learn Valerie's name. But I would never say any of this in front of Julian.

"This has been special, Mark," I said. "You are a dear and special friend."

We sat in our little circle on the grass under the apple tree. Shadows darkened the lawn, the mountains clouded over, the cove turned green-gray. I felt as if we should all hold hands, but we didn't. I reached out and wiggled Julian's toes. Then I punched Mark in the shoulder.

"Remember when ..." Mark launched into a reminiscence about our crazy days together. And we fell over laughing. "And remember when ..." We laughed more, giggles and belly-twisting laughing, rolling-on-the-grass, stoned, mellow, wide-open laughing.

"Chicken's ready," Valerie called from the porch. And we went in to eat roast chicken, rice, and ratatouille with fresh zucchini from their garden.

Ingrid Bergman, Gregory Peck, and Julian

On Thursday, Julian and I went to see two old Ingrid Bergman films at the Stanford Theatre. Julian loves Ingrid Bergman. He idolized her when he was a kid. So when the Stanford Theatre had an Ingrid Bergman festival of her movies, he was thrilled. We discussed our outing the night before, that morning, and that evening over dinner.

Driving down University Avenue, I saw a long line outside the ticket booth. "Get out," I told Julian at the corner of Emerson and University. Gesturing toward the crowd, I said, "You get in line and I'll park the car."

I parked several blocks away and returned to the theater. Julian was not outside the theater, nor was he waiting for me in the lobby. The movie had already begun.

"Did a gray-haired man with a beard leave a ticket for me?" I asked the ticket-taker, explaining the situation. "I'm sure he's in there," I repeated, persuading him finally to let me enter.

Inside the darkened theater, I waited in the aisle until my eyes adjusted to the blackness. I searched the rows for Julian's familiar curly hair. Still no Julian. Up on the screen, Ingrid Bergman was driving recklessly in a convertible down a palm-tree-lined boulevard, with Cary Grant sitting next to her. She was drunk, her hair disheveled. Cary Grant wore a dark suit and tie, and his hair was meticulously combed and slicked down despite the car's speed.

I scanned the left side of the theater, where we usually sit. No Julian. I went out one door and in the other to scan the right side. Ingrid Bergman, still sozzled, was now letting Cary Grant into her apartment. She flopped down on a sofa. Julian wasn't on the right side either. Too many people sat in the center section for me to find him there. The theater was packed. So I sat down and watched the film, figuring I'd find him after it ended. Cary Grant was persuading Ingrid Bergman to spy for the U.S. government on some ex-Nazis in Rio.

After the movie the crowd left the theater. Still no Julian. I stood outside the men's restroom, watching each man exit. I whistled our "family whistle": "da doo da doo." I asked a man going into the men's room to call Julian's name. My mind formed a backup plan: (1) Look down the street in Cafe Fornaio and the Prolific Oven. (2) Drive home. See if he's there. (3) Phone the police.

Suddenly, Julian appeared in the lobby, gray hair tousled, his face glowering. I walked toward him, relieved to see him.

"Where the hell were you?" he barked. "Why didn't you wait for me? Why'd you go off and leave me? You just walked away. I waited for you."

"No, Julian," I argued. "Remember, I went to park the car. Remember, I let you out to stand in line while I parked the car?"

"You left me," he hissed. "I was standing right here." I explained again. Standing red faced near the water fountain, I explained and reexplained. "Remember we came to see Ingrid Bergman?"

It turned out that Julian had gone to the Aquarius Theatre just around the corner and seen *Daughters of the Dust*.

"Don't you remember we came to see Ingrid Bergman?" I insisted.

Just then I understood. Julian had gotten out of the car at the corner of University Avenue and Emerson. While I had looked at the line outside the Stanford Theatre and gestured toward that crowd, he had been looking down Emerson at the Aquarius, in his direct line of vision.

No point arguing. No point continuing to try to get him to understand. He was only getting angrier and more irritated. He had paid for two tickets at the Aquarius; I had gotten in free to the Stanford.

"Never mind." I laughed and took his arm. "Let's go see the second feature." Julian pulled his arm away, stiffening his body against me.

We entered the darkened theater. This time Ingrid Bergman was wearing a white medical coat and large eyeglasses. Her hair was pulled severely back in a tight bun. She was a psychiatrist at a posh mental hospital. Gregory Peck, the new director of the institution, entered the doctors' dining room.

I reached over and took Julian's hand. He pulled it away and tucked it under his leg. He wouldn't hold my hand. He shifted away from me in his seat. Gregory Peck and Ingrid Bergman ate lunch in the dining room and left for a ride in the country. Julian got out of his seat and soon returned with a box of licorice. He handed me five hard, sweet little bits of candy. Gregory Peck had an anxiety attack after seeing Ingrid Bergman's striped bathrobe. Julian kept handing me licorice.

When the candy was finished, Julian took my hand. My hand felt warm, safe, and familiar in his. At the movie's end, Ingrid Bergman had solved Gregory Peck's neurosis, explained the mystery of his panic attacks whenever he saw stripes, and cured him of his amnesia. And Ingrid Bergman and Gregory Peck got married and lived happily ever after.

Turning Time

September 21: the autumn equinox.

A friend and I have come up to Silver Lake to see the aspens turn. Willow bushes flanking the beach near our cabin are turning yellow, pale gray-green leaves interspersed with gold. Across the lake, golden aspens shimmer against deep green firs behind. There's a nip in the breeze although the September sun is still warm. The day lasts as long as the night. Starting tomorrow, nights get longer.

Fall 1992

It's the turning time.

Next week is Rosh Hashanah, the Jewish New Year. According to tradition, we must assess our lives during this past year and prepare for the coming one. We review our thoughts and actions, deeds and inactions.

Modern Jews have re-phrased the Orthodox long list of transgressions. "Grant me forgiveness," they say, "for my sin in polluting the air and the water, in speaking ill of my neighbor, in failing to act." There's plenty to consider.

Supposedly we have ten days to reflect before the coming year. On Yom Kippur, the day of repentance, God stamps and seals our fate. On this awesome day it is determined who shall live and who shall die, who shall die by fire and who by drowning, who by illness and who by stoning. The possible ways of dying go on for pages.

Of course, I don't believe that God stamps and seals our fate. But the ancient words linger, reminding me of the uncertainty of our lives. They recall loud and clear that we are all destined to die and no one knows how or when. Our life is temporary and precious. We are each headed toward the end. Only the timing is unclear.

The prayers also say that on Yom Kippur it will be determined who shall live in bitterness and who in peace, who shall dwell in envy and who with acceptance. Between Rosh Hashanah and Yom Kippur, we are blessed with the opportunity of choosing. We can turn away from what we don't want and turn toward what we do want.

It's the turning time.

The water level in Silver Lake is at its lowest these last days of summer. Waves lap gently on the stony beach, near jagged hunks of black volcanic rock, usually concealed by water. Across the cove, aspens quiver, orange and yellow, crimson and chartreuse. It's quiet this Monday of the autumn equinox. Families have returned to school and work, weekenders to the cities. Warblers and chickadees have flown to warmer places; chipmunks and squirrels gather seeds for winter. It's the end of summer, the turning time.

How do I wish to turn?

I want to turn away from fear toward acceptance. If I truly accept Julian at each moment and stop expecting him to be different, then perhaps I won't feel so irritated and afraid. I want to stop needing him to be as he used to be. I want to be able to let him go. My helplessness and inadequacy cling to him, preventing me from acceptance. I want to trust myself to handle whatever comes. I want to move from sadness into joy, to collect all the joyful moments I can and store them, just as chipmunks around our cabin gather seeds for the cold ahead.

A sharp wind lashes the waves. A chill in the air bites at my skin. Summer is ending. The time of resolving, changing, and doing is upon us.

It's the turning time.

"Happy New Year. Love, Julian"

I rummaged through my desk drawers and found some Rosh Hashanah cards not sent in previous years.

"Let's write the New Year's cards tonight," I said to Julian after dinner. It was our first night home alone together in ten days. I had been in the mountains for a week, then came a stream of dates and activitites. Now Rosh Hashanah had just passed.

"Perfect," I said. "We'll write short notes to the Glasgow and Israeli families. Mail them tomorrow. And they'll get them by Yom Kippur."

"I don't like them to go . . . be there . . . you know . . . write before . . . after the day . . . you know . . . not the time . . ."

"I know," I said. "You like the cards to arrive before Yom Kippur. It's okay" And I whipped out a piece of paper and listed the names. "You write a short note and I'll add a few lines, too." "Don't write a whole letter. Just say 'Happy New Year—Love, Julian' or 'Wishing you a healthy and happy New Year.'"

I knew Julian's brother and uncles in Glasgow and his sisters-in-law, nieces, and nephews in Israel would feel relieved to see his handwriting, confirming that he's still okay. Of course, they worry. I gave Julian a pile of cards and the list.

"I want to write a proper letter," he said, rejecting my suggestion of writing a simple greeting, and he disappeared into his study.

An hour went by. A second hour. I addressed twelve envelopes and wrote twelve short messages. About two and a half hours later, Julian emerged from his study holding a single sheet of lined paper.

"It's so hard to write," he said. "Now I'll copy it over."

He no longer trusts himself to write freely. Now he makes rough drafts first. He had written his brother in Glasgow, and he showed me the letter. At first glance I was pleased to see a full handwritten page.

But as I started to read it, it didn't make sense. Sentences started off and ended in an ungrammatical, nonsensical stream of unconnected words. Words were scratched out and rewritten. His handwriting sloped down the page, not remaining on the lines. Yet it was unmistakenly Julian. No simple "Have a happy New Year" for him. He was still trying to write originally and say something unique in his own special way.

My heart sank. I remembered how shocked I was a year ago trying to help him edit a story for his autobiography class. Then, the language was simple, the paragraphs were in a strange order, and events were sometimes out of sequence. There were only occasional misspelled words; this man prided himself on his impeccable grammar and spelling and clear, excellent command of English.

But this letter shocked me further. This is Julian, I reminded myself. This *is* how he is. It's his letter to his brother, written with love, the best he can do. I thought briefly of not sending it, of discouraging him from mailing it, as I knew it would upset his brother.

The family in Scotland is less used to handling things in the open. An institutionalized, retarded niece is never mentioned. His mother wasn't told she had cancer. "Let's not tell anyone else," his brother wrote when I first told him about Julian's Alzheimer's diagnosis, two years ago.

I remembered when my toddlers started dressing themselves and put their T-shirts on backward or inside out. Or when they wrote in big, printed letters, spelling words phonetically exactly as they sounded. I treasured their efforts. I didn't correct them. It was the best they could do.

Well, it's the best Julian can do, too, I told myself. Of course he should send his letter.

Julian sat with me at the kitchen table copying his letter onto a clean page. No point trying to correct it. Too many words were misspelled and hardly a sentence made grammatical sense. Why shouldn't his brother see him as he is?

But when Julian showed me the copied version, I was shocked again. He couldn't even copy what he had written. One sentence started off and was never completed. Fragments appeared at the bottom of the page. He was unable to look at the original and remember a few words long enough to transfer them to the new page. Or to track his place on the line.

I didn't cry. Didn't gasp. Didn't comment. I just added my note, folded the letter and sealed the envelope.

"Kenny'll be glad to hear from you," I said. "He'll be happy to get your letter."

Only partly true. Kenny will be glad to hear from Julian, but he'll be shocked and saddened to receive this evidence of his brother's decline. Should I have shielded this from him? Or should I simply let things be, as they are?

I printed clearly, "Happy New Year. Love, Julian" on a slip of paper.

"Here, darling," I said. "Add this to the cards I've written." And I showed him the space on each card where he should write. Maybe the nieces and nephews will treasure these messages one day. I felt oddly distant and accepting that night as we wrote the cards.

But all the next day, I was irritable and downhearted, even though nothing in particular had happened.

Losing the Toyota

I was sitting on the sofa, curled up under an afghan, drinking tea with a friend, when Julian opened the front door, talking loudly

Fall 1992

with another man. It was five o'clock, gray and raining outside. Julian was home early.

"I found Julian wandering around by the museum," a familiar voice said, and Gig, a longtime colleague of Julian's, entered the family room with Julian behind him.

"So I gave him a ride home," he said.

"But where's our car?" I asked, puzzled. Julian had taken the car this morning because it was pouring rain and because his bike had been stolen the day before, as he had forgotten to lock it.

"I left it . . . I left the car . . . over there . . ." Julian began explaining, looking sheepish and flustered.

"I didn't mean to make life more confusing by bringing him home," Gig said. "I was only trying to help."

Gig knows about Julian's Alzheimer's, I'm sure, through the professional grapevine, though I've never discussed it directly with him. I can tell by the extra friendliness with which he greets us these days when we pass him on the road or meet him in the market. The increased jolliness says between the lines, "I know. I know."

"I can take you back to Stanford to get your car," my friend Eileen said, finishing her tea.

"I have to get home or I would take you myself," Gig said.

"No bother," Eileen said, getting up.

After Gig left, Julian said, "But . . . the car . . . I put it on the ground . . . I don't know where . . . I couldn't find it . . . when I called you before, it was already lost."

Julian had phoned me midafternoon, as he usually does, to check in. He explained that he had already been searching for the car for two hours but he didn't tell me because he didn't want to upset me.

"Never mind," I said. "Eileen is just leaving and she'll take us back to get our car. We'll drive up and down the lanes of the med school parking lot. We'll find it. No big deal."

The three of us got in Eileen's car. As she drove toward the medical school and Julian's office, Julian kept saying, "You don't understand. It's not there. It's far away. It's not in the parking lot . . . it's not at Stanford . . . I put it on the ground . . . I just left it. I don't know where I left it. I don't know why I left it. But I stopped and got out. I don't know why I did that. I got out and walked around. I didn't know where I was and then I couldn't find it and it's over there . . . far away . . . not at Stanford . . . by that brown place . . . north . . . up north . . . way up there . . . by a brown place . . . I put it on the ground . . . where people live . . ."

"Was it near your office?" I asked.

"No, no . . . people live there. . . ."

"A dormitory?" Eileen said. "An apartment building?" I guessed.

Eileen and I bombarded Julian with questions. I hoped to retrace his movements from where he had last been with the car to where he was headed. As Eileen circled the parking lot, she questioned him on the physical description of the place he had last been. Our questions only confused him.

"No, no," Julian said. "Not here . . . far away . . . not on campus . . . a brown place . . . a tight place . . . a not wide place . . ."

"A narrow place?" I asked.

"Yes, narrow."

"You couldn't turn around?"

"Yes . . . no . . . it was narrow. It was a brown place. People lived there."

Eileen drove around the medical school, past Julian's office, and to the buildings beyond. We drove up and down the streets adjacent to the med school looking for our white Toyota station wagon with half of a ski rack, which we keep attached to help us find our car in parking lots.

By then it was dark. Streetlights and headlights glistened on wet slick streets, the roads congested with Stanford employees going home from work. We decided to quit and search again in the morning.

Eileen dropped Julian and me back at our house and went home. Julian took a shower. My hands trembled as I boiled pasta and poured a jar of marinara sauce into a pan, suddenly feeling terribly alone with a disoriented man.

I had never seen Julian so confused or flustered. I had never heard his language break down like that. I felt a cold clutch of fear in my throat. I thought of the men in the Alzheimer's group who had gotten lost: the man who drove around the Bay Area for two days trying to get home from his daughter's house and the man who drove to the market and ended up in L.A. We'd been lucky. Only the car was lost, not Julian.

Advice sheets handed us by the VA Alzheimer's and Memory Disorder Clinic said, "All memory-impaired people will eventually get lost, sooner or later." But it was Julian's confusion that scared me, not the lost car. Could I handle this full-time, I wondered. "You poor dear," Eileen whispered to me before she went home. "I had no idea."

Julian returned from the shower, wearing his pajamas and maroon bathrobe, his curly gray hair dripping. I brought the pasta into the family room and placed it on the coffee table. We ate and watched *Mystery*, our favorite TV program, as if nothing had happened. I sat close to Julian on the couch. I ruffled his hair. After dinner I stretched out and wiggled my feet in his lap. He squeezed my toes. He seemed calmer. His language settled down and full, logical sentences returned.

"I'll not take the car again," he said, though later he would not remember saying this. "I'll manage on my bike. I don't know what happened to me."

The next morning we borrowed Eileen's car and retraced Julian's trip from the Food Closet in Palo Alto, where he volunteers on Thursday afternoons, back to the medical school. I hoped that retracing his trip would jiggle some memory of where he had gone or where he had left the car.

"It's far away," he kept saying. "It's by a brown place . . . I left it on the ground . . . it's where people live . . . it's way up. . ."

I kept guessing: "Is it on the campus? In Palo Alto? In Menlo Park? In a residential neighborhood? By an apartment house?"

No use. No car and no clarity either.

"I'll drop you at the bike shop," I finally said. "Buy another secondhand bike and I'll notify the police."

At the Stanford police station I described what had happened. A tall, moustached, uniformed officer listened sympathetically and took notes on a small pad.

"We'll search the campus tonight when there are fewer cars," he said. "And on the weekend. If we don't find it in twenty-four hours, we'll notify the Palo Alto and Menlo Park police."

I drove Eileen's car back to her house and she drove me home. I called the Stanford police every six hours at the change of each shift. Forty-eight hours later, as Julian and I set the table for breakfast, an officer announced cheerfully, "We found it."

"Where?" I said.

"In a cul-de-sac on a little side street on campus about two blocks from the med school." He gave me directions.

Leaving Julian at the table, I pedaled my bike to the location the officer had described. I had never worried about the car; I knew we'd find it. But seeing Julian so unable to express himself was a glimpse of the future. I thought of more confusion to come. Will I be able to comfort him, care for him, keep him happy and safe? Will I be able to accomplish this and maintain some sort of meaningful life for myself? Will I be able to keep on loving him?

I followed the officer's directions and turned left off the main campus road onto a little side street which I had never noticed before. There, parked in a regular parking area, in front of a maintenance building, was our white Toyota, sitting in full view of the med school, not two blocks from Julian's office.

Hoisting my bike into the car and driving home, I realized that Julian had just gone straight on where the familiar Campus Drive curved slightly. He had stopped on a dead-end street flanked by strange buildings. His internal map isn't yet gone, but it's going. Anything unfamiliar is enough to confuse him.

Even the significance of familiar items around the house can baffle him. This week I've seen other signs of perceptual confusion. He often brings me his razor and his toothbrush, asking which he should use to brush his teeth—a perfect example of the agnosia Nancy Mace described in her lecture. When I said yesterday we needed a "paper clip" to clip some papers together, he looked at me blankly as if I had spoken Chinese. "Paper clip?" he asked, puzzled. "What's that?" Words suddenly lost meaning—a different kind of agnosia, this time for words.

This morning he complained he had no clean socks and I told him to look in the dryer. When I entered the kitchen, he was rummaging through the dishwasher.

"I can't find them," he said. "My socks aren't here."

"This is the dishwasher," I said, then led him into the laundry room. "Here's the washing machine. And here's the dryer."

We opened the dryer door. "Voilà! Clean socks!" I said triumphantly as Julian looked at me sheepishly.

Back home, I entered the kitchen and found Julian drinking coffee. "It's okay. I've got the car."

Julian looked up at me and smiled.

"You're my darling man," I said putting granola, yoghurt, and bread on the table. "My darling man." A year ago I would have been furious. But I'm slowly learning to accept what can't be helped.

I took a deep breath, sighed, and sat down to eat my cereal. Julian pedaled off to the library on his newest bike (to be lost before the month was out). And I drove off (gratefully) in my white Toyota to accomplish this day.

Martial Art

Parents and children settle themselves in chairs set around the YWCA's activity room. A dark-skinned toddler sits on the lap of her blond mother. An Indian-looking little boy holds his red-headed father's hand. Caucasian women sit next to African-American men, while children of different hues run about the room.

My daughter, Karen, and her husband, Beiçola, an African-Brazilian martial arts instructor, walk to the center, ready to demonstrate Capoeira, in which Beiçola holds a Rio de Janeiro championship.

Beiçola stands in the circle, dressed in his white cotton pants and white sweatshirt with the logo of his Capoeira school silk-screened on the front. A wide grin stretches across his dark face as he tells the crowd how Capoeira began in Brazil when the Portuguese held Africans as slaves. He raises his leg and demonstrates a kick, telling us that Capoeira is a martial art done to music, a mix of singing, dancing, powerful kicks, and turns. A game, a fight, and a dance.

My slender daughter, fair-skinned and blue-eyed, stands behind Beiçola, dressed in the same white uniform. She softly beats out a rhythm on a maroon drum as Beiçola speaks. Karen has been doing Capoeira since she was twelve. Their six-year-old son, Antar, sits cross-legged on the floor beside her, in an identical uniform, next to three other boys.

I sit in the front row with Celina on my lap. Her black wavy hair, pulled into two bunches on top of her head, tickles my chin when I bend to whisper in her ear. Her cocoa-colored hand rests in mine, and I'm aware of the beautiful contrast in our colors. Her tiny Capoeira outfit lies draped over my knees, but she shakes her head when I ask if she wants to put it on and do Capoeira with Mommy, Daddy, and Antar. Julian sits next to us, studying the California motor vehicle guide. He's been called down to the DMV to take a driver's test tomorrow.

Karen, Beiçola, and Antar are demonstrating Capoeira for I-Pride, an organization for interracial couples and families. The Y is offering a Capoeira class taught by Beiçola's friend, who has invited them to this presentation.

Karen beats the drum while Beiçola explains that when the blacks were slaves in Brazil, they weren't allowed to gather in groups for fear they might revolt. So they created simple drums and one-string gourd instruments. They played music, sang, and "danced," or so the Portuguese slave owners thought. In reality, they were developing kicks and turns, practicing ducks and dodges that appeared to be a dance, while they were actually training for a fight.

Karen lifts the gourd instrument, strums the string, and, to its twangy sound, sings in Portuguese. Beiçola starts moving slowly to the music as he speaks. In slow motion he demonstrates forward kicks, back kicks, and deep dips to the floor. He turns one-handed cartwheels and stands on his head, first with his legs pointing straight up and then angling his body off to one side. Slow, so slow. His biceps bulge as he stands on one hand, his powerful body motionless in the air. All the while he smiles and laughs. Soon the audience loosens up and smiles too.

Beiçola beckons Antar to "play" Capoeira with him. Antar, his dark head barely reaching Beiçola's waist, cartwheels out into the game He kicks, twirls around, does a back kick at his dad. Beiçola grins and stands on his hands, smiling, singing, and laughing as he spins and kicks, gentleness and warmth in his controlled strength. Suddenly he leaps up and flips over backward, landing on his feet. The audience gasps.

The music picks up speed. Beiçola invites the other boys to play. He gets the audience to clap the Capoeira beat. My hands slam together in the familiar rhythm. Celina on my lap is clapping. Julian puts down the DMV manual and claps too. Everyone is clapping: the moms and dads, big kids and toddlers, the incredible rainbow of different faces, all smiling.

Soon Beiçola has half the audience standing in a circle tentatively imitating the basic steps. Karen plays the drum, singing and chanting. When I get up, Celina slides off my knees and climbs onto Julian's lap. He folds his arms around her and kisses the top of her head as she snuggles into his embrace. I walk into the circle and join the novice group. We kick forward, then back in the basic pattern.

One by one, Beiçola invites each person into the circle's center to play Capoeira with him. Smiling and laughing, he encourages us to attempt the movements. A man in a business suit loosens his tie and squats down in the starting position. A woman in a flowered skirt and silk blouse slips off high heels, giggles, and attempts a kick. Beiçola has softened this crowd and made them enthusiastic. A tiny, thin, brown-skinned girl twirls around, clutching her bottle.

Beiçola beckons me into the center. I know a little Capoeira, as I took his class last summer for four weeks and actually earned my beginner's belt. I get into the rhythm of the basic step and do my best forward kick. Pretty good: a one-breasted, fifty-three-year-old Jewish grandmother with arthritis doing an Afro-Brazilian martial art. I even turn a cartwheel, to the left, my good side, as I can't do cartwheels at all to the right.

Playing Capoeira totally absorbs me. Gone are the worries I came in with: Julian's driving test tomorrow at the DMV (when he'll probably lose his license), his lost bike, his lost briefcase, the lost VCR tapes of his autobiography (probably in the lost briefcase on the lost bike). Gone are my frustrations over this morning's conversation—who's going where, when, and what's happening at what time (each statement needing to be repeated and clarified in excruciating detail). Gone is the memory of yesterday's talk with a woman from the Alzheimer's couples' group (when I learned that one husband became sexually abusive and was put in an Alzheimer's unit at a nursing home, another is now tranquilized because he became unmanageable, and a third has died).

Here I am at the Y, doing my kicks and turns, awkward and clumsy, but I'm playing nonetheless. My leg kicks out at my gorgeous son-in-law, who dodges, twirls, leaps, and grins back at me. Karen beats out the rhythm; Celina sits on Julian's lap, the two of them clapping. The DMV manual has slid to the floor under his chair. Antar plays another round of Capoeira with his dad.

Our birthday dinner for Beiçola waits at home on the already-set kitchen table festooned with the fresh flowers Beiçola loves. I am here at the I-Pride workshop, filled with pride for our family: Karen, Beiçola, Antar, Celina, and Julian, each clapping, smiling, and laughing.

"Yay Capoeira . . ." sings Beiçola.

"Yay Capoeira . . ." we all sing back, clapping our hands to the irresistible beat.

Listening to a Heartbeat

Friday night Julian and I met my sister and brother-in-law at a restaurant in San Francisco to discuss my dad's housing dilemma. The four of us sat around a square table—white cloth, linen napkins in large water goblets, fresh flowers—and ordered calamari sautéed with capers, Caesar salad, and a good chardonnay. We exclaimed how delicious the calamari was and how reasonable the prices.

Then we began discussing my father.

Fall 1992

My dad is in a financial crisis. At eighty-one, still recovering from his neck cancer surgery and having recently had his tracheotomy tube removed, he's just learned he has no money. He has exhausted his savings, will get no more money from a marital trust he's depended on, and must leave within two months the pleasant retirement home that he loves.

I tell my sister that I've submitted three applications to low-income, federally subsidized housing in the area, the only ones with waiting lists of less than a year. The other retirement housing for seniors has waiting lists of two to five years. My sister tells me she's submitting an application for assistance in reducing Dad's health costs. The medical application packet is two inches thick. I tell her I've written letters to the lawyer managing the trust, the director of Lytton Gardens, the illusive housing of our choice, and to the executor of the trust, in a last-ditch effort to get the money.

I think of my dad with the small white bandage in front of his neck, which covers the gaping hole from his tracheotomy, which is slowly closing. I think how his voice is regaining its usual baritone quality, how the watery gurgle is disappearing. I think of his Halloween costume, an African outfit given him by a student from Kenya, which he'll wear to the Halloween party at the retirement home next week. He deserves to be comfortable, to enjoy himself and stay in a place he likes.

My sister and I plan our strategy for the next weeks: She'll call the county courthouse and make an appointment to get the court records. I'll write the executor of the trust and call Lytton Gardens to see if special circumstances can improve his placement on the waiting list. I tell her I'm taking him to the ear, nose, and throat surgeon and his internist for follow-up appointments next week. Julian and my brother-in-law sit quietly eating their calamari while my sister and I talk. Over hazelnut flan and decaf, we scan the senior housing book one more time to see if there are possibilities we may have missed.

The wedding starts at eleven o'clock on Saturday morning. Julian and I sit in the third row in Stanford Memorial Church. The well-dressed crowd files in, filling row after row of wooden pews. The daughter of a speech therapist friend of mine is being married. I sit next to Tom, a pediatrician we both worked with in a clinic twenty years ago, when the bride was a toddler.

The church's gold mosaic ceiling glistens. Blue, red, and yellow stained-glass windows depict scenes from the flight from Egypt and the stations of the cross. The wooden dome is freshly polished, the church festooned with flowers, the organ softly playing.

Tom leans over and whispers, "What are you doing tomorrow afternoon?"

"Oh," I say. "Don't ask. I'm going to a memorial service for my good friend's husband who dropped dead of a massive heart attack four days ago. I'm helping her arrange the service, get food, flowers," I whisper back.

"Someone else has died," he tells me. "I'm going to a memorial service too. Romayne died yesterday."

"Oh, no," I say. "Oh, no. Not Romayne."

Romayne was a woman we had both worked with at the clinic. She was exactly my age and had had a mastectomy just a few weeks after mine. Like me, she had also had positive lymph nodes and chemotherapy. We had talked on the phone. I had sent her my cancer poems. I had just seen her a few months ago and she looked fine. How could she be dead?

Suddenly the organ plays some loud chords and people scurry to their seats.

"She developed bone cancer and went downhill fast," Tom whispers. "She died in the hospital of complications from chemo."

Suddenly here comes the bride's mother, my friend, walking proudly down the aisle in a pale green silk suit. Ten bridesmaids in bright crimson suits walk—step-pause, step-pause—down the long aisle to form a wide arc before the altar. The ushers, tall, lanky young men in black tuxedos form a curve on the other side. Julian and I watch the wedding party take their places.

The organ shifts to "Here Comes the Bride," that tune that brings tears to my eyes even when I don't know who's getting married. And here comes the bride, yes, all dressed in white satin, her hair covered by a flowing veil, on the arm of her father.

Fall 1992

Bride and groom stand before two ministers, one wearing a white robe, the other black, flanked by the ten bridesmaids and ten ushers.

"Do you take this man to be your wedded husband . . ." the minister in the white robe asks. ". . . to have and to hold, from this day forth, for better, for worse, for richer, for poorer, in sickness and in health, till death do you part?"

The bride, so young, so sweet, softly answers, "I do," staring into the eyes of the tall, slim youth before her.

I think about those vows as the minister repeats them to the groom. I slip my right hand into Julian's, my left hand reaches out and rests on his arm. He's wearing his brown tweed sport coat, his dressiest jacket.

"I do," says the groom. It's all so beautiful, this pageant, these weighty words so easy to say.

The wedding party troops back down the aisle to the triumphant chords of the processional. Outside the church, under the arches of Stanford's quad, guests stand around and mingle before driving to a luncheon in a nearby restaurant.

I'm not going to the reception, as in half an hour I'm speaking in a workshop called "Gay and Lesbian Youth: The Hidden Minority in Schools." I'm to be on a panel with Stanford students and a father of a lesbian daughter. I'm there to tell my story as the mother of a gay son. The workshop is part of a day-long conference for psychotherapists called "Sex, Love and Family."

Under the arches I see another speech therapist I worked with twenty years ago, a slender, gray-haired man who had been the director of the clinic. He had recently been treated for a cancerous growth. We had talked during his convalescence. I had sent him my cancer poems and he had told me how much they meant to him, even though they were about breast cancer, a mastectomy, and chemo, and he had had surgery and radiation on his arm. The fear and journey toward acceptance is nearly the same.

Bob and I catch sight of each other and fly into each other's arms. We hug, a long, tight embrace. The joy of surviving sparks back and forth between us.

"Your poems meant so much to me," he says. "Let's sit together at lunch."

"I'm not going to the reception," I say.

And I tell him why. I tell him I am active in Parents and Friends of Lesbians and Gays because my oldest son is gay. It all rushes out. I haven't seen Bob for years, and only recently did it occur to me that he is gay, too. So I blurt out about my talk that afternoon on gay youth. And he hugs me again. We kiss each other many times, currents of affection present in each kiss.

In the gay and lesbian workshop, I sit behind a long table with others on the panel. The moderator tells the audience of therapists that approximately one third of youth suicides are gay and lesbian. He tells of the fear, anxiety, and loneliness most gay and lesbian youth experience as they wrestle with coming to accept their orientation.

An eighteen-year-old Korean Stanford student, an African-American lesbian sophomore, and a Chinese-American youth speak before me on the panel. They describe their struggles in high school to accept being gay in a world of negative stereotypes, inaccurate information, and no positive role models.

When it's my turn, I speak for ten minutes. I tell my story — how Ben told me he was gay, how I felt then, how I feel now, and how I moved from being afraid and ashamed to the work that I presently do. I tell them Ben is a wonderful, happy person in my life.

Several people in the audience brush away tears. Afterward two students on the panel throw their arms around me and give me big hugs. "Thank you," the Korean boy says.

Sunday morning, just before I leave to help my friend prepare her house for the memorial service, another friend from Berkeley calls. Her mother's ninety-fifth birthday was yesterday. I didn't go because of the gay youth panel. She wants to tell me how happy her mom was: ninety-five years old, in good health, her mind bright and alert, a wicked Scrabble player, the matriarch of our seders. Karen went to the birthday, representing our family. She videotaped Esther, surrounded by children, grandchildren, and great-grandchildren, cousins and friends, listening to her grandchildren say how much she's meant to them, what they've learned from her, how she's given them strength. The grandchildren cried, my friend tells me. Esther ate her birthday cake, enjoyed the flowers, and heard the stories, totally there.

At Joe's memorial service, Eileen's and Joe's friends fill the living room. They sit on the couch, the love seat, the piano bench, the ottoman, and folding chairs. White snapdragons lean out of a blue vase on the piano. The dining table, covered with my white lace cloth, holds platters of fresh fruit, bagels, cream cheese, and smoked salmon, a cheese board and crackers, banana bread and cookies. Flowers, food, friends—all the ingredients of a party, but the host isn't here. He collapsed four days ago on a sailboat and died. He cannot hear the stories, laugh with his friends, and eat this good food. Everyone says how much he would have liked it.

I thought of Esther, who reigned yesterday at her party. I looked over at Julian sitting on the ottoman, still so alive. He's warm and breathing and cuddly. It occurs to me that as fast as Joe died, that's how slowly Julian is leaving. But he's not gone yet.

In bed that night, I lie next to Julian, his warm body wrapped around mine. The weekend's events flash before me: the discussion about my father's housing; Saturday's wedding of the so innocent bride and groom; the intensity of feelings on the gay and lesbian panel; Esther's ninety-fifth birthday and Joe's memorial gathering.

I feel my heart thudding. Tears fill my eyes. I can't sleep. The richness of this weekend keeps me awake until long into the night. I press closer to Julian and squirm until I fit perfectly into the curve his body makes. I lay my head on his chest and feel the thud-thud, thud-thud of his heartbeat.

Singing Hallelujah

"Hallelujah . . . de da da . . ."

I don't remember the words to this prize winning Israeli song, but its tune has filled my head for days.

Julian's practiced it for hours, preparing for last night's performance of the Yiddish Chorus. He played a tape of the rehearsal over and over, learning the words. He had his secretary type the words in a large font, as it's too hard for him to read the small printed sheet music. He retreated into his study all weekend to sing along with the tape.

Last night the Yiddish Chorus sang at the Jewish Community Center's Hadassah meeting for the installation of new officers. Julian and I went. I accompanied Julian because I was afraid that if he went alone, he'd get lost and arrive late. Or turn the wrong way going home and end up in Portola Valley in the dark and be unable to get back.

It seemed too complicated to ask him to return the video we had rented to Blockbusters, which would involve coming home from the Center an unfamiliar way, and then to pick up Ben from his job at the Country Sun on time or meet him at the bookstore if he wasn't there by ten. All this was too difficult to explain and too much to worry about. So I decided it was simpler to go myself.

And besides, I love the Yiddish Chorus! I love Julian's singing in it and the happiness it brings him.

Julian wore his required black pants, white shirt, and tie. He had put on his new black leather shoes, purchased the day before as an attempt to help his arthritic toes. He looked terrific. So handsome to my eyes, his curly gray hair, his freshly trimmed beard. He looks like a rabbi these days as he gets older, or a pious Jew, especially when his glasses slip down his nose, especially when he's in the Jewish Community Center.

The Hadassah meeting was boring beyond tears (though I certainly understood it was for them, not me). A hundred well-dressed matronly women sat on folding chairs listening to the praises of out-going officers and the backgrounds of incoming officers, interspersed with snippets of Biblical lore about Moses and Sarah and facts about Henrietta Szold, the founder of Hadassah. I wrote a letter. Julian shuffled his music pages, putting them (again) in the right order.

Periodically I eyed the long table of cookies, cakes, and bagels laid out on the white tablecloth beside me.

How did we end up at a Hadassah meeting anyway? Julian would have avoided such a gathering two years ago. He would never have spent an evening this way; nor would I.

But now we relaxed into it. Gone were the relentless pressures to read the latest physiology research literature, write an NIH report, or review grant applications, the never-ending demands of his career and his choice of how he wanted to spend his time. Now Julian feels a relentless pressure to enjoy life. He feels an urgency to do new, easier, and enjoyable things.

"Smile this time," I whispered to Julian, who focused seriously on arranging the music. "You're here to have fun. It's not an exam," I said. "If you don't know the words, just hum, or go 'la-la-la.' Or stand there. No one will ever know if you're singing or not. Enjoy yourself."

He's always worried that he won't be able to sing the words fast enough.

The chorus marched up to the front of the hall. Julian stood in the back row, looking down at the music a lot, but singing and smiling. He caught my eye and grinned. He looked so cute up there happily singing these songs of his youth.

The chorus sang old Yiddish songs by Molly Picon—"*Yiddle mitn Fiddle*"—and Hebrew songs—"*Hallelujah*"—and songs his father and grandmother sang in Poland and Russia. Tears filled my eyes.

A tall gray-haired woman with gnarled arthritic hands accompanied the chorus on the piano, and a guitarist and trumpet player added pizzazz. The chorus sang, slightly off key but with enthusiasm and verve. The audience clapped and sang along; I joined in tapping my feet.

"I love this," Julian said to me as I drove home. "I don't like that other place, where I feel diseased."

He meant the Alzheimer's Couples' Group we attended at the Veterans' Hospital two days ago.

"I feel sick when I go there. I feel like I'm sick," he said. "I don't want to feel like I have a disease. I just want to live my life."

"Hallelujah . . . de da da . . ." I began to sing in the car. Julian joined in. We sang "Hallelujah" all the way down Arastradero Road to El Camino to return the video, and back up El Camino to California Avenue to pick up Ben.

"Hallelujah . . . da da, da da da . . ." filled the car.

A day later the "Hallelujah" tune still runs through my head.

Julian Is Honored

Julian and I were in bed, reading the newspaper and sipping our tea, when the telephone rang. I answered it. It was Manuel Mas calling from Spain.

"The ceremony is set for the last week in November," Manuel said in his Spanish accent. "Come a few days early for the rehearsal. Send us Julian's curriculum vitae, a scientific biography, and a fifteen-minute speech on the significance of his work. And fax us immediately his head size, ring size, and measurements. Tomorrow you'll get a fax listing exactly what we need."

Excitement and fear swirled together in me like marble cake.

Manuel Mas, a doctor in the Canary Islands and a colleague of Julian's, had arranged for the Universidad de la Laguna to grant Julian an honorary degree. Last year Manuel's medical school had sent Julian an elaborately decorated diploma shortly after Julian's diagnosis. What superb timing, when Julian's career was plummeting along with his self-confidence and self-esteem.

Manuel's university's president had written Stanford's president and the dean of the medical school. They, in turn, wrote Julian letters of congratulations. A tribute to Julian's career, just at the time he was having to let it go.

"The ceremony was scheduled for January, but they've moved it up to late November," Manuel said. "That's in one month. We'll need the measurements right away and the bio and speech by next week."

I gulped, my head swimming with visions of Julian marching in an academic robe to receive his degree in a formal pageant. I thought how much this would mean to him, how much fun it would be to look back on and remember.

Then I thought of Julian trying to read a speech, much less write one. Anxiety took over.

"It'll be hard for Julian to do that," I cautiously said to Manuel. I couldn't go into details, as Julian was right beside me in bed. "A fifteen-minute speech?"

"Nobody will understand," Manuel said. "Very few speak English. And I'll stand next to him. I can even help him write the thing."

Julian took the phone and spoke with Manuel. He got up out of bed and paced up and down the hallway as he talked, the way he always moves about when talking and excited.

Conflict churned within me. On the one hand, what a wonderful tribute to Julian. He deserves to have his life's work acknowledged. On the other hand, what if he gets confused? Can't read the speech? Or marches the wrong way in a formal procession? It might be fun or it might be disaster. But Manuel knows how Julian is. He visited us this summer. He knows Julian's language is awkward, his comprehension poor.

"We'll have to protect him," I had said when we'd discussed the possibility of this ceremony last August.

"We'll sit next to him at the dinner," Manuel said "And surround him at the reception."

But what if he breaks down and can't read the speech at all? What if he says silly things or gets lost in Tenerife? What if he can't answer when a professor speaks with him?

What if . . .

After Manuel hung up, Julian and I talked. Did he really want to go? Was it worth the money for my ticket? Could he write and deliver a speech? Or could someone help him write it? Maybe someone else could read it? I slept little that night. Excitement and anxiety kept me tossing and turning.

The next morning, when I was alone, I phoned Manuel in the Canary Islands.

"We want to come," I told Manuel. "But I'm afraid. I don't want Julian to embarrass himself or you. He's more confused than when you saw him last summer. It's impossible for him to write a speech. He can't write a coherent letter to his brother. I doubt if he could even read," I said, remembering just this morning Julian's laborious reading of a few sentences from the morning paper. He read slowly and with great effort, stumbling over and mispronouncing words.

"We'd have to help him," I said. "Someone would have to write the speech and probably read it. Maybe you? Maybe me?"

I wanted to go, but I was afraid. My fear rose up. But my sense of adventure rose too. Crazy to pass this up because of my anxiety. I felt a surge of confidence in being able to handle potential problems.

"If you understand the situation," I said to Manuel, "we'd like to come."

"Good," Manuel said.

"Let's go for it," I said. "Maybe you could just tell them Julian's had a stroke or laryngitis and can't deliver his speech," said my worry self. "Let's just do it. As long as we can protect Julian and keep a sense of humor."

As Manuel spoke, questions tumbled in my brain. The really big one surfaced: What should we wear? Julian doesn't even own a suit. The dressiest he can get is corduroy pants and a brown tweed jacket. And what should I wear? My usual garb is pants, a turtleneck, and Reeboks. I needed to phone the travel agent and start checking on tickets. Whom could I ask to write Julian's talk on the significance of his work in behavioral endocrinology?

"We're coming," I told Manuel. "We're coming."

A Desperate Daughter

Walking down the beach, I watch the orange disc of the sun slide into a metal-gray sea. Shiny, hard sand turns gold. Sandpipers scurry and avocets run after each receding wave, poking thin beaks into bubbling sand.

Fall 1992

Suddenly I come upon the sandcastle. A deep moat surrounds thick walls topped with turrets. A long ramp slopes up the east side. Circular towers festooned with seaweed flags protect each corner; bits of broken sand dollars and crab shells decorate the castle walls. Tunnels through arched doorways lead from the outer rampart into the keep.

Buckets, cans, and shovels used in its construction lie scattered on the sand. A crowd of sunset walkers gathers to admire this extraordinary castle. Children point and exclaim, their skinny bare legs protruding from baggy sweatshirts. Two mothers take photographs. Placing my hand on a damp wall, I marvel at its thickness: firm and cold under my pats. A few grains of sand trickle down. . . .

Yesterday my friend Eileen called and asked if I would go to the post office with her to pick up her husband's ashes. Two days ago she had received the little yellow paper in the mail.

"I'm afraid to go alone," she said.

"Of course I'll come," I said. And I drove over to her house. Her husband, Joe, had collapsed of a massive heart attack two weeks earlier on their vacation in Florida. His body had been cremated and the mortuary had sent the ashes by certified mail.

I thought of Joe the last time I had seen him: sitting at a round table at Printers Inc. doing the *New York Times* crossword puzzle and drinking a cappuccino while Eileen and I talked.

"They say bits of bone and teeth stay in the ashes," Eileen said as I drove to the central post office. "I don't know if I want to open the box or not."

"Look or don't look," I said. "Do whatever you feel like doing."

I parked, switched off the ignition, and turned to look at her—white faced and small in the passenger seat. I made no move to open the door.

"I miss him most in bed," she said. "Not just sex. But rolling over at night and touching him. Holding him. Feeling his warm body next to me. Sometimes I dream about him. I dream he's alive and I wake up excited and happy. Then I remember he's dead and it's like learning he's gone all over again."

I settled in the driver's seat and adjusted my legs to a more comfortable position.

"Did I ever tell you how I met Joe?" she asked. And she proceeded to tell me how she felt when she met him and how she had left her husband and he had left his wife so that they could be together. She poured out an intense, passionate, and turbulent story.

"I've never told this to anyone," she said. She described how hard Joe had been to live with and how she loved him.

She said, "He was a difficult man, but I got everything I wanted. I've been deeply loved. I have no regrets."

Inside the post office we stood in a line waiting for the next available window. A young Asian man said, "How can I help you?"

Eileen handed him the yellow notice. He took it, disappeared into a back room, and returned with a small box wrapped in brown paper, about eight inches long, four across, and four deep, smaller than a shoebox. Eileen lifted the parcel from the counter.

"Oh, it's heavy," she said.

"Have a nice day," said the clerk.

Eileen cradled the box in her arms like a baby, and I put my arm around her waist as we walked to the car. She sat in the passenger seat and I got into the driver's seat and we just sat there. We didn't speak. Eileen held the box on her lap. Tears filled our eyes in the long silence. After a while I reached over and lifted the box.

"It *is* heavy," I whispered, surprised at its weight.

As I drove home she continued her tale. We sat outside her house in the driveway in the car while she talked.

"I've never told all this before," she said again.

I just listened. When it was time for me to leave, I said, "Eileen, thank you for sharing this time with me." I told her how many of our days just slip away and blend one into another, forgotten. But not this one.

Fall 1992

"I'm okay," she said, getting out of my car and carrying the box down her driveway and into her house.

That night my daughter phoned as I watched the evening news in bed. Julian was already asleep, the newspaper still in his hands, crumpled on his chest, his glasses low on his nose.

"Mom, Mom," Karen cried, sobbing so hard I couldn't understand her rush of words. "I have to leave, Mom, I have to leave," I heard.

Calming down and stifling her sobs, she told me a car was on fire near her house on a dead-end street near the freeway in Richmond, an hour and a quarter away from Stanford. A fire engine and three police cars were parked outside her window, their red lights flashing. Her husband was in France giving Capoeira workshops and wouldn't be back for a month. She has felt uneasy in that neighborhood these past weeks. She has already told me of a drug-related murder two weeks ago and how recently her six-year-old and his friend found a pistol under a van.

Then she said a neighbor, also watching the burning car, told her a man had been prowling around her house the night before, peering into her windows.

"I can't stay here, Mom," she cried. "I can't stay here!"

Dad and I will be right up, I immediately thought. But what good would we be? Julian couldn't think straight in any emergency, and I felt as afraid as Karen.

"Go to a friend," I said. "Right now. Or I'll call my friends in Berkeley and you can stay with them."

"I have to move, Mom," she sobbed. "I can't stay here. It's not safe. My children aren't safe!"

"Hang up, Karen, and call Susanna." Susanna is her friend with children the same ages as Antar and Celina. "We'll make a plan. Call her now."

Julian woke up and shoved the newspaper onto the floor. "What's happening?" he said.

Solutions raced through my brain: whom I could call, where they could move, how we might finance it.

Alzheimer's, A Love Story

I thought of Antar, representing his first grade class in student council, finding a gun. I thought of his best friend on the block, whose mother's boyfriend is an addict. I thought of the halfway house for drug rehab on the corner. I thought of Celina, sleeping in her bottom bunk under her Little Mermaid quilt.

I thought how Karen loves that house. How Beiçola had painted all the walls before they moved in and had painted the trim on the doors and windows lavender. How for three days he had sanded and waxed all the hardwood floors.

I phoned Karen. "I'm going to Susanna's," she said. "She has a studio cottage in her garden. I'll stay there at night until Beiçola gets home."

I sighed, relieved that Karen and the children were safe for now and would be okay until Beiçola returned. But her words echoed: "Crazy people on drugs with guns are near here, Mom. My children aren't safe."

And my child's not safe. All night I tossed and turned. Could they move to a safer neighborhood? Could they afford to buy another house when they can hardly manage the payments on this? The life they've worked so hard to create is threatened. You get your act together and suddenly the fragile props are knocked away. It's all so precarious. . . .

The next morning, when I opened my eyes, Julian stood by the bed holding the phone. It was Manuel from Spain saying he had received all the faxes—the measurements, the bio, and the speech which was written by a friend. It's all done. We've nothing more to do.

Julian stood in his underpants, a long-sleeved white shirt, one hiking boot with the laces trailing, and one black tennis shoe.

"I need to send him . . . tell him . . . you know . . . the notes I've been reading . . ."

"You mean writing?" I asked.

"The material . . . I need to add . . . that he wants . . . I must tell him . . ."

"Manuel says everything's handled," I said. "There's nothing more to do. We just have to go there."

But Julian couldn't let go of feeling he needed to do something. He couldn't comprehend that everything was done. All that day and that night he wanted to call Manuel.

"But you talked with Manuel this morning," I said. "Remember? Manuel called today. There's nothing you must do."

As we sat at the breakfast table over coffee and granola, we discussed the day. I was to meet Julian at the house for lunch. Then we would both drive to Richmond to visit Karen for the afternoon. Then I would babysit the kids while Karen taught Beiçola's Capoeira class. And Julian would have dinner with his good friend Irv. Then we'd drive home.

But he couldn't get it. He got confused. I told him over and over, trying to stay calm. I wrote the appointments in his calendar, which he tries to keep in the fanny pack I've finally convinced him to wear. I wrote it down on a piece of paper.

"First, lunch," I wrote. "Then Richmond. Then dinner with Irv. Then home." Over and over I repeated what we would do that afternoon.

Sipping my coffee, I then jotted down what I had to do that morning before we left:

1. Go to the police station and have them sign off Julian's citation (that he got two weeks ago for driving without a license and not finding the car registration).
2. Go to traffic court with the signed citation.
3. Send photos of Julian by Federal Express to Manuel in Spain.
4. Go to the DMV to hand over Julian's revoked driver's license.
5. Take my dad to the ENT doctor.
6. Make an appointment for Julian at the podiatrist.
7. Phone Julian's secretary about the autobiography tapes.

The list continued. Obviously I couldn't do all this today. "To Do" I printed at the top of the page and got up to get a second sheet. No sooner do I run to one problem and try to fix it, than another develops. Staring at my list, I kept thinking about the sandcastle. . . .

I remembered that evening, walking back up the beach. Orange streaks shone on glistening gray sand, and black clouds covered the darkening sky. The sea rose and fell, white froth sliding up and back. I came again to the sandcastle.

It stood alone in near darkness at the edge of the surf, its builders and admirers gone. Waves slid up the slope, filling the moat. One wave, stronger than the last, hit the western wall, which crumbled, trickles of sand slipping down, forming dark brown mush.

I scooped a handful of cold, wet sand and shoved it against the wall, patting it back into place. Around the corner the southern wall began sliding too. I crawled to that side of the castle and pushed sand up that wall. The sand gave a thudding sound as I slapped it.

As soon as I strengthened one wall, another started to slip. I couldn't keep the walls in place, no matter how fast I worked. Finally I turned my back to the castle and walked away from the black sea toward the lights of distant houses, quickly, without looking back, before the next wave came.

The Loss of Independence

Julian and I enter the conference room of the VA Alzheimer's and Memory Disorder Clinic, happy to see only two other couples. Helen, the facilitator, waves a welcome as we pull two chairs into the small circle.

The "New Couples' Group" met three times last spring, but it didn't meet all summer. Helen starts our session by asking whether we find this small group helpful and whether she should continue it or whether the large couples' group meets our needs.

"The other group is important," I say quickly. "But for me, it's too big. Thirty people is a lot. You often don't get a chance to talk. Only the spouses speak. The people with Alzheimer's don't participate. And also, they're in more advanced stages."

I don't tell Helen how frightened I feel in a room with fifteen Alzheimer's patients in more advanced stages. I don't say how painful it is to listen to talk about day care, sitters, respite homes, night wandering and pacing. I have enormous sympathy, believe me. We'll be there one day, too, I suspect. From the group I learned about coping, about courage, resilience, and love. But it was too depressing for Julian, and he stated clearly that he wanted to stop. I continued a few times on my own, but now I've stopped too.

"Yes," the others in the group agree. "It's too big. We can all talk here in this smaller group."

"So, how are things going?" Helen begins.

A thin, tentative, gray-haired woman named Jane says,"I get so confused at times. I move slowly. I think slowly. Tom gets mad at me."

All eyes watch Jane as she speaks. She's wearing faded jeans, white tennis shoes, and a denim shirt, a silver Medic Alert bracelet on one wrist, a watch on the other. She twists her wedding ring as she speaks.

"Things take longer when you have memory problems," Helen says. "It takes longer to think. You must allow more time to think what you're going to do or what you want to say. Be patient with yourself and give yourself lots of time."

"But I'm a one-two-three kind of guy," her husband says. He is tan, bald, with a fringe of gray hair; he's wearing a yellow Izod shirt. He tells us he's arranged for people to come in and stay with Jane so that he can run errands and have time to play golf. A home companion comes Mondays, a cleaning woman on Tuesdays, their grown granddaughter on Thursdays.

"I just feel pushed around," Jane says. "Everyone tells me what to do all the time."

Helen speaks slowly, validating Jane's feelings and encouraging her to say what she feels. The group nods as she speaks. The other Alzheimer's patients tell her they feel these things too.

"And how are you, Julian?" Helen turns to him and asks. Julian pours out the story of how his driver's license was revoked last month and he doesn't understand why.

"What did I do wrong?" he asks for the hundredth time. "I've never had an accident. I think I drive okay. I'm very careful."

Helen has explained many times during the past year how Alzheimer's affects driving. She has specifically told Julian on several occasions that Alzheimer's affects reaction time.

"People with Alzheimer's process things slowly," she says again. "They need more time to read and interpret road signs, street names, and signals. Driving is complicated. It involves processing many things at once. You have to react quickly. Many things come at you fast, requiring quick decisions."

I glance at Julian's face as she speaks. He's watching her, listening intently. I pray he gets it this time.

"It's not that you can't physically drive the car," she says. "You can still handle the mechanics of driving. But people with Alzheimer's get lost if their usual freeway exit is closed. Or if they have to take a detour. They become disoriented if something unusual happens.

"It's a big loss of independence," Helen adds gently. "Not driving causes changes in every family. It's a loss that takes a long time to accept."

"Yes, yes," says the stocky man sitting next to me. "I lost my license a year ago and I still feel bad. Before that I had to stop flying." He had been an airline pilot when Alzheimer's forced him to retire. "It's hard not being able to jump in the car and go where I want to go."

Each person with Alzheimer's tells how they came to stop driving and how they feel about it. Each spouse describes how it affects them too.

"And you, Ann?" Helen nods to me.

"Well, we have good news and bad news," I begin. "The good news is that we're leaving for Spain in three days, as Julian has been awarded an honorary degree in the Canary Islands."

"That's wonderful." Everyone smiles at Julian.

"The bad news is, as Julian said, that he lost his license and he's having a hard time accepting it."

Helen explains again in her slow, calm voice. She says how difficult it is to let go of independence and that safety is important. Julian watches her and listens.

"I understand," he says. "But why couldn't the DMV explain instead of just jerking my license away? Anyway," he adds, "I have my bike."

"Another thing worries me," I continue. "Just before his license was revoked, he lost the car, for forty-eight hours, on the

Stanford campus. Eventually the police found it. I never worried about the car. But Julian was terribly upset. I've never seen him like that. I was frightened. He was confused and disoriented. He couldn't explain what happened, where he had been, where or why he left the car. He was agitated and his language fell apart."

"Sometimes," says Helen slowly, "people have what we call a 'catastrophic reaction,' if they're under stress or if they're in an unfamiliar place and suddenly don't feel safe. This happens when people get lost."

"Yes, yes," I say. "It was raining hard that day. He left the car only two blocks from his office, but he got totally confused."

"Things look different in the rain," Helen says. "That's enough to make him lose his way."

I feel relieved hearing this explanation. I had been scared that Julian would remain in that incoherent state. But I also realize with deeper understanding my role in being organized. I must do everything possible to anticipate problems, arrange, and plan to minimize stress. I know all difficult situations can't be avoided. If things sometimes get out of control, it isn't my fault. But I have a large responsibilty to keep life calm. I vow to be more alert so I can head off problems.

"I'm also worried about our trip to Spain," I say. "We have three long flights with three-hour layovers in international termi-nals. And Julian's having a hard time letting go of the fact that he doesn't have to 'do anything' in the Canary Islands, except enjoy himself. It's hard for him to let one colleague write his speech and another read it."

"It's hard to let go," Helen repeats in her quiet voice. "Living with Alzheimer's involves a continual need to adjust. It's hard not being able to do things you're used to doing. It's hard having to ask for help." She looks right at Julian, who lowers his eyes.

"As for the trip, don't try to do too much in one day," she says. "This is true for regular life too. Do half of what you usually do. Leave plenty of time for transitions. Double the time you usu-ally allow to prepare to go somewhere. Have unscheduled slack time to rest."

Jane's husband is writing notes on a yellow pad. I see him write "allow time" on his paper and underline it.

"Jane broke a glass in the kitchen yesterday," he says. "She wanted to clean it up, but I didn't want her to cut herself so I told her to go upstairs and take a nap and I would clean it. Then she got mad at me. All I did was want to help her."

"Can anyone think how they might handle that differently next time?" Helen asks.

"He could have let her clean it up or they could have swept it up together," the stocky man says.

"Yes," says Helen. "Independence is the issue. People with Alzheimer's have to depend more and more on others to help them. No one likes to feel helpless and dependent. So anytime a person can do something themselves, they should, even if it takes longer or isn't done efficiently."

I am touched by Jane's sweet hesitancy and how relieved she looks hearing her feelings acknowledged by Helen and the group. I'm moved by her husband's blunt desire to help her and his willingness to learn how to handle things more easily. I am relieved myself to have my worries understood and to get suggestions for how to manage.

Our hour is up. No one wants to leave. We have each spoken. Our fears and upsets have found the right ears: Others understand and nod their heads. Yes, yes. Helen, wise and experienced in dealing with Alzheimer's, makes suggestions. I feel more confident about our trip.

"Have a wonderful time," everyone tells us. "It's a marvelous honor for Julian," Helen says. "Enjoy yourselves. I'm sure the trip will go fine."

We stand up and say our goodbyes. "I'll send out notices when the small group meets next," says Helen.

"Good, good," everyone says. I look from Jane to Tom to the stocky man to Julian. Their faces look more relaxed than when they entered. I know my face feels softer and my shoulders have sunk down an inch. It feels so good being heard.

Off to Iberia

They've turned on the cabin lights and announced that it's morning. "*Buenos días, señores y señoras, seis y medio en la mañana,*" I hear

[114]

over the loudspeaker. Middle-aged stewards in dark, pin-striped suits bring us coffee and juice. "We'll be landing in one hour and twenty minutes."

I'm in my bleary, blotto phase. It's hot and stuffy; I can't get comfortable in this prison of a middle seat; my throat is dry. I had just fallen asleep (eight P.M. California time), and now it is morning.

In the past twenty-four hours, Julian and I have had two fights, embedded in an otherwise pleasant trip. Ugly as they were at the time, they ended quickly. For this I am grateful. In the old days—the old, healthy days—we had fights that could last for hours. But I let go of irritation quickly now. I can't seem to control its flash and rise, but I can control what happens later. I can apologize, take deep breaths, be quiet for a few moments, and resume. How many more pleasant hours I would have had in life had I learned this sooner.

One fight erupted last night at home, sitting in our kitchen eating leftover pasta before scurrying around to do last-minute packing. Earlier that afternoon Julian had driven the car back to his lab for some forgotten items. His license had already been revoked. But still he took the car even though he had said he wouldn't. He began shouting when I reminded him he shouldn't drive.

The second fight exploded a few hours ago at Kennedy Airport at a hot dog stand in the middle of the international terminal during our three-hour layover.

"I can't stand this," I ended up yelling at him. "I'll never travel with you again. Go travel with somebody else!"

People at adjacent tables turned to stare. Then I got up and stomped down a wide corridor, leaving a bewildered Julian sitting at the white plastic table with a sad, hurt look on his face. I only walked a few yards, keeping him in sight by glancing over my shoulder. I walked as far as a trash bin, where I threw away my crumpled napkin. Then I walked back.

I sat down again at the white plastic table. "I'm sorry," I said. "I'm sorry I yelled. I lost my patience. That will happen sometimes. Now it's over."

Julian's mouth turned down like a forlorn child's. He wasn't ready to let go. What had happened? I hardly know. Nothing really. But whatever it was, I had felt that hot surge of irritation. Frustration at not being understood and not understanding him. Anger at no longer having an intelligent companion. Sadness at what's become of Julian.

We were sitting at the hot dog stand, cheerful and congenial after a pleasant flight to New York, when Julian began talking about where he wanted to go in Spain. He asked me repeatedly how many days we'd be there, when the ceremony would happen, when Ben and Jeff were coming—even though we've been over this many times. Then he began:

"I want to go over there . . . up there . . . over there . . . to that big place . . . not that other place . . ."

"You mean you want to rent a car and travel around the island?"

"The big place . . . that other place . . . up there . . ."

"You mean Spain? We aren't going to Spain itself. We're going to the Canary Islands. We can travel around on the island."

"No, no . . . up there . . . the other place . . . where I was . . ."

And so it went. Around and around. I couldn't make myself clear to him and I couldn't understand him either. I thought he was still talking about wanting to travel in Spain or Portugal after the ceremony in Tenerife. I had vetoed that idea when I bought the tickets. Just when I had been making the plans, Julian had lost the car, had had his "catastrophic reaction" and become terribly confused. Then he had his driver's license revoked. I was afraid to travel alone with him in a foreign country where I don't speak the language and where he might suddenly become disoriented. In normal times, of course, we would have. I liked nothing better than being alone with Julian in an exciting new place. But no more.

Perhaps I was grieving over our lost independence there in the airport. Just when we have the time and money to travel, we're unable to do it. It's enough of a challenge to fly to the Canary Islands and back. Maybe I was feeling a rush of that remorse. But I wasn't patient. I didn't sit quietly and let him talk. I felt irritated.

"Tenerife is an island," I said. "There's water around it. We

can't go to Spain. Our ticket is just to Tenerife and back." I
snapped out simple sentences over and over which he didn't
understand. And he got stuck on some endlessly repeating loop
where I couldn't understand what he was trying to say.

In the quiet of this writing, I see all I had to do was to sit
calmly and listen to him. Just let him talk and try to understand.
I shouldn't have persisted in trying to make him understand me. I
didn't need to explain. I didn't need to be "right" or have him see
it my way. But it's hard in the heat of the moment.

So I ended up screaming, "This is the last trip I'll ever take
with you!"

Five minutes later we walked arm in arm down the corridor
to the departure gate.

"You know I love you," I said. "I'm proud of you. Only it's
hard for me to be patient all the time."

"You make me sick when you talk to me like that," he said.
"You talk to me like I'm diseased. Like I'm some kind of terrible
creature!"

"I'm sorry," I said. "I am truly sorry."

We've had minor ruffles before. Julian hadn't brought his
fanny pack. At the last minute, he left his wallet and calendar at
home, in which I had carefully written all the flight information
and dates of different events. Julian was walking around three
international airports headed for Tenerife with no wallet, no I.D.,
no awareness of where he was going. He refuses to wear the
Medic Alert bracelet with his name and address engraved on it
which I ordered for him months ago.

I watched Julian fumble. I watched the steward look at him
blankly when Julian tried to ask for juice. I watched him unable
to answer "coffee" when the steward asked "Coffee or tea?" Julian
could not produce the word "Coffee."

"Keefa," he tried. "Feeca."

I watched Julian try to fill out the landing card. Only four
items were requested: surname, first name, birthdate, where the
passport was issued. Julian stared at the card. He couldn't figure
it out. He signed his full name in the middle of the card, not on
the clearly designated space. He had no idea what information was

requested. I showed him my completed card. He copied "3-3-38," my birthdate, onto his card.

"That's *my* birthday," I said. "Write in yours."

He paused. He shoved his glasses up on his foreheaad and thought and thought, head in his hands.

"When's your birthday?" I asked.

Silence.

"April fifteenth," I said. "Write 4-15. Do you know what year?"

Pause. Embarrassment. I could have told him outright. But I am curious about what he does and doesn't know. It helps me understand what to expect. He didn't know the year. Finally I said, "1931. You were born in '31."

This is the man I am traveling with. I need to know.

The trip so far has been smooth. With these exceptions, it's been pleasant. Only I carry the tickets, the passports, the traveler's checks, the itinerary, my purse, the day pack, our coats. I don't trust Julian to carry one thing. I can't let him out of my sight. I find men's and women's rooms adjacent to each other and we go to the lavatory at the same time.

"I'm just led around like a puppy," he says.

But Julian is more docile and cooperative than he was last year when we traveled to Scotland to visit his family. Then he still thought he was independent, and we struggled over who would carry the tickets. He insisted on carrying his passport, resulting in frantic searches through all his pockets each time it was needed. This year he lets me carry everything without a fuss.

Now we're flying over Portugal en route to Tenerife. Maybe we should have gone to Portugal while we are here. We've come so far. We have the time. But would it be fun to travel alone with Julian in a new country when I don't speak Portuguese? When the trip goes smoothly, I think maybe we can. Maybe I'm being overly cautious.

But when I see him not know his birthdate, ask me what "gate" means and what "those white things down there are called," I know my decision is right.

"Clouds," I tell him. "Clouds, my darling. We're flying over the clouds to Tenerife."

Life Through a Second Lens

Julian and I have been on Tenerife two days; I'm watching the scene through different lenses. The first absorbs the sights: high, blue mountains rising out of an aqua sea . . . the bare rocky hills we passed while driving from the airport along the south coast toward the capital city of Santa Cruz . . . the broad, palm-tree-lined boulevard approaching Manuel's wife's office . . . a demitasse of espresso and hot milk—a *cortado*—drunk while perching on stools in a crowded cafe. . . .

Sitting with Manuel in a country restaurant on the side of a hill sloping down to the ocean, eating garbanzo beans and chorizo, large barbecued squid, cubes of goat cheese, and long, thin white sweet potatoes. Visiting the medical school and Manuel's office, where Manuel pointed to a chart on the wall picturing androgen functions and the hypothalamus, put out by a drug company. Manuel showed me Julian's work cited four times in the reference section.

But I view all this through a second lens too. Julian is on the periphery. He rarely speaks. I try to be quiet and let him converse with Manuel. Manuel delivered interesting facts about Tenerife as we drove along, but Julian didn't respond. So I make comments and ask questions, and the conversation keeps sliding over to Manuel and me.

Manuel took us to his white stucco home with a red tile roof and a white wall surrounding the garden of which Maria is so proud. Bushes of red, yellow, and white hibiscus, geraniums, poinsettias, bougainvillea, and birds-of-paradise filled the courtyards. From their patio you look directly at a 12,000-foot volcanic peak, the Teida, towering above banana plantations in the valley below.

Then Manuel drove us to our hotel, a white tiered structure of balconies and terraces with pink and red geraniums hanging from flower boxes on each level, three turquoise pools, and a view of the sea. Manuel ushered us into our two-room suite with white tiled floors, white furniture, and a balcony overlooking Puerto de la Cruz, six kilometers down the coast.

That first evening, Manuel and Maria picked us up at nine-thirty to drive to Puerto de la Cruz for what was to them an "early" dinner. We went to their favorite restaurant in a two-hundred-year-old Spanish house, enthusiastically ordering baby squid in garlic sauce, calamari, Spanish mushrooms.

Only Julian didn't order. He said he didn't feel well and went to the men's room. He never returned. Manuel made four trips to check on him, but Julian said he felt sick and needed to sit there. As we'd already ordered the food, the three of us ate our meal and talked.

Manuel asked how Julian was. I said he had changed since last summer when they had visited. He's much more confused. Now, just over two years since his diagnosis, he has trouble reading even simple notes with comprehension. He can't write three correctly spelled, grammatical sentences. I told them he lost the car one block from his lab. Tears welled up in Maria's eyes as I spoke. My voice warbled and caught in my throat. Maria took my hand.

After dinner Julian returned to the table looking pale and said he needed to go back to the hotel. Maria put her arm around his waist as we left the restaurant. Her jolly laughter rang out as they walked arm in arm to the car. On the drive home Julian slumped down in the backseat and went straight to bed as soon as we reached our room.

Today Julian feels weak, so we're taking it easy. We have the whole day to ourselves. We ate breakfast in the hotel dining room. Then we took the bus into Puerto de la Cruz and walked along the seaside promenade — past Cafe Columbus displaying three-layer cakes in the window, past huge turquoise swimming pools with white deck chairs filled with sunburned tourists speaking German, Swedish, and Dutch.

Julian carries no wallet, no money, no calendar, no I.D., and no notepad on our sight-seeing jaunts. He has no concept of Spanish pesetas and makes no effort to learn. He doesn't know the name of our hotel or even what town we're in. He follows me sweetly and doesn't dash away to look at things as he did in the past. He sits down often on wooden benches in the shade of white buildings. We're enjoying the scenes and our carefree stroll, but it occurs to me that my companion is rather like the sweet, near-sighted, confused, cartoon character Mr. Magoo.

I look at tourists passing us on the promenade: most are gray-haired couples, probably retired, and I marvel at the competency of these older men. They talk freely, follow maps, convert money, add up their change, calculate tips, and can find their hotel. Julian can do none of these things.

But saddest of all is that it's so difficult to talk to Julian, except for the most concrete, immediate remarks.

"Look at that black sand."

"See those jagged volcanic rocks?"

"Look at that fabulous chocolate cake. Let's bring Ben and Jeff here when they come on Tuesday."

He continues to ask when the boys are coming, where Manuel is today, and when the ceremony will take place. I've written the facts on a card, including Manuel's phone number and our hotel address, which I've put in his pocket.

Will I ever accept not talking freely with Julian? It's easier when we're walking past interesting sights to point out and comment on; it's hardest when we're alone together over a meal. He misunderstands much of what I say, even if I restrict myself to only simple sentences. He can hardly produce a sentence without word substitutions, the words sometimes not even semantically close. He says "food" when he means "book," or "drive" when he means "eat." I must decode what he says. I can understand him best if I already know what he's talking about or if I know the context.

Last week, back in Palo Alto, a woman in the Alzheimer's group told me, "I so miss talking with my husband!" And her husband is competent enough to take the train alone into San Francisco to spend the day!

Today, sitting on a bench by the seaside promenade, near a park festive with bougainvillea, geraniums, and hibiscus, near a wall where two green parrots perched, Julian looked at me and suddenly said, "I love you so much. I love you with my whole heart. What would I do without you?"

I took both his hands in mine, my eyes moist with tears, regretting my recent thoughts of Mr. Magoo. How unfair to think that way. Those thoughts push me away from Julian, when what I want is to feel close while I can.

At the pool this afternoon, I watched a slender young couple splash and tease each other in the water, the electricity between them unmistakable. They emerged, dripping, from the pool and lay side by side on two white chaise lounges. He stroked her thigh. She ran a finger down the dark, wet hairs on his chest. He rolled over and kissed her. She removed his glasses. They lay on their sides facing each other, kissing again and again, then left and went to their room. I imagined them as honeymooners and remembered all the zipping and unzipping of our early urgent love.

It's now nearly two A.M. Julian went to bed hours ago. He put on his maroon pajamas, said "G'night," and went to sleep. Out beyond our balcony, the lights of Puerto de la Cruz sparkle under a black sky at the edge of a dark sea. Orion's belt hangs in the darkness and there shine the Pleiades. Music from a wedding in the hotel dining room drifts in through the open window.

I write this now, lying on the flowered sofa in our sitting room while Julian sleeps in the bedroom next door. I wear my pale blue nylon pajamas and I can't sleep. The air feels chilly. I put on Julian's beige windbreaker over my pajamas to keep me warm.

A Chorus in Latin

The first day on Tenerife, Julian and I visited Manuel's house. Manuel ushered us into his study to view the academic gown he and Julian will wear in the ceremony: a long black robe with yellow satin cuffs covered with lace and a yellow satin hood and mantle. He showed us his white leather gloves. Then he held out a high domed hat with yellow fringe that looked like a lampshade. As he placed it on his thick, black hair, we burst out laughing.

"Manuel, you look like a lamp," I said.

"Julian will get a hat like this too," he said.

"Two lamps." We all laughed.

Julian tried on the yellow hat and pranced before the mirror. Then Manuel showed us the book published for last year's honorary professors. The slick volume contained a color photograph of each, his acceptance speech printed in Spanish, and a list of his publications. Photographs showed the university president slipping a ring on one gowned professor's finger and placing a gold chain with a medallion over his head.

"It's an elaborate, sixteenth-century academic ritual, and I must study the protocol for the ceremony," Manuel said. "As Julian's sponsor, I will make a proposal speech describing his contribution to science."

Julian stood in Manuel's study, the lampshade hat tilted jauntily to one side.

"There's only one more thing Julian must do," Manuel said. "Read this." And he handed Julian a paper, three quarters of a page printed in Latin.

"*Ego* Doctor Julian Mordecai Davidson," it began. ". . . *iuro quod honorem, reverentias, commoda, et praeminentias huius almae regis sancti ferdinandi universitatis canariarum . . .*"

Julian roared with laughter. He stumbled over a word or two, then dissolved in giggles. I tried a line, struggling to recall my junior high school Latin. "How do you pronounce this word, '*idemque*'?" I asked Manuel. "And '*quocumque*'?"

Manuel took the paper and read in a sonorous bass the ancient words, sounding like a priest chanting the Mass. "Just read the first and last lines clearly and mumble the middle," he suggested. "Probably few people in the audience will understand Latin. It doesn't matter if you pronounce the words correctly or not."

But Manuel didn't really understand that Julian could barely read English, much less Latin.

In our hotel room that night, Julian began practicing his Latin. At first he laughed and mumbled loudly, pretending to be a priest. But then he began studying it silently and underlining the longer words. His face grew solemn. "I'll practice and practice," he said. "I have four days to learn it."

"How do you say this?" he asked, pointing to "*magistrarumque*" and "*praeminentias.*"

He read and reread the Latin text in his spare time over the next two days, in bed at night before turning out the light, and sitting on the white plastic chair near the geraniums on the balcony in the sun. I read it aloud several times myself, but I always broke down somewhere in the middle, either from laughing or from my tongue refusing to twist itself around the long, unfamiliar words.

"Just read the first line clearly and mumble the middle," I repeated Manuel's instructions. "Then read the last line clearly."

But I began to worry. If Julian couldn't read it here quietly in our hotel room, how would he be able to read it during the ceremony with an audience's eyes on him? I didn't want him to embarrass himself or Manuel by breaking down and coming to a humiliating halt.

"You know this memory thing . . ." Julian said the third day after lunch. "No matter how many times I read a word, I can't remember it. This memory thing has destroyed me. Look at this," he said, showing me a long underlined word.

"No matter how many times I practice it, it doesn't get better. A regular person could learn and improve. I can't."

Still the scientist, I thought, observing and analyzing behavior. Those who think that people with Alzheimer's don't understand what's going on are very wrong.

"It's going to be awfully boring for the audience to hear the Latin oath four times, if each honorary professor reads it by himself," I finally said to Manuel on Sunday as he drove us along a twisty, narrow road atop a volcanic ridge toward the northeastern point of the island. The blue Atlantic stretched on three sides off into the hazy horizon. "Maybe all four could read it together?" I suggested. Manuel looked thoughtful.

Over plates of tiny fish and slices of calamari and potato croquettes, Manuel asked Julian, "Can you see without your glasses?"

Manuel had told me earlier that Maria's idea had been to tell the people planning the ceremony that Julian had lost or broken his glasses and that was why Manuel would be reading Julian's speech.

"Can you see that tree over there, for instance?" Manuel was concerned that if Julian removed his glasses, he wouldn't be able to see the ceremony.

My idea had been for Manuel to just tell the planning committee the truth, that Julian has some "neurological problems" that prevent him from reading. Or that because he and Julian had a binational grant and had collaborated on research projects, he would read Julian's speech in Spanish so that the audience would understand.

"But Manuel," I said, squeezing lemon on my calamari, "if Julian supposedly can't read his speech because he's lost his glasses, then how can he read the Latin oath?"

Silence fell over our group as we pondered this dilemma. Maria and Manuel talked rapidly in Spanish. "We'll work something out," Manuel said.

In the car driving back to our hotel, Maria tried the Latin. She couldn't get through it either. I tried again. Maria, Julian, and I roared with laughter. Only Manuel could read it. Our son Ben, long active in theater productions, could do it. Maybe when he arrived on Tuesday, he could teach Julian. Maria and I held our stomachs laughing on the balcony while Manuel tried to coach Julian in our room.

"Seriously, what do you think about the four professors reading the oath as a chorus?" I repeated as we said good night to Manuel and Maria in the lobby of the hotel. Manuel had to go home to write his speech that night and study the ceremony. "It's a possibility," Manuel said. "Let me think about it."

Later that evening, just before Julian and I turned out the light, the phone rang. It was Manuel.

"Good news," he said. "I phoned the protocol director and he said a chorus of four professors reading together would be just fine."

"Whew." I let out a long sigh. And Julian left the Latin oath out on the kitchen table and didn't practice it in bed that night.

Finding 89-B

Our room number in La Quinta Park Hotel is 89-B. You exit the lobby toward the swimming pool, walk the length of the pool, descend two flights of stairs and turn right. On the first level, numbers 102–92 are posted on a sign with an arrow indicating turn right; numbers 91–81 are posted on our level.

We've been here four days and Julian still hasn't learned the location of our room. I've shown him, verbalized the directions, and indicated landmarks. Still he doesn't know. Each time we return to the room, I let him lead the way and he makes a wrong turn at every place where there's a choice. It's taken him days to orient himself to even find the stairs. He wanders about the pool somehow unable to recall that one walks away from the lobby and passes the pool to get to the stairs.

Even as he descends the steps, he ambles off at every level but our own. Sometimes higher, sometimes lower. When he does turn off, it's invariably left instead of right. Then he can't remember "89-B" and continues walking past our door.

When I point out to him the little sign on each landing giving the range of room numbers, he looks at me blankly. It's hard even for him to follow my pointing finger to see what I'm indicating. When I ask him if 89 falls between 102 and 92, he looks puzzled. He has no idea.

"Does 89 come between 102 and 92?" I ask him, sounding like his neurologist asking who the president is during a mental status exam.

I remember back two and a half years ago when we went to an international endocrinology conference in Acapulco and later traveled in the Yucatan peninsula. On that trip I first realized something was very wrong with Julian. He lost his lecture notes and slides at the airport. Although he read his talk okay, he was unable to answer questions from the audience. A doctor asked him a question after his presentation, and Julian looked blank. The man repeated the question and Julian answered, "You're absolutely right." I couldn't understand why he did that.

Later, as Julian and I traveled for a week in the Yucatan, I became aware that he never learned to pronounce the names of the Mayan ruins: Uxmal, Chichenitsu, Palenque. I didn't know how to pronounce them at first either, but I learned. Julian didn't. He was confused in each hotel as to where our room was, and he never found his way in each new town. I took to carrying the keys, holding the map, leading the way. I handled the money and calculated the exchange rates. It just sort of happened. I might not have noticed these changes in Julian for several months had we not been traveling in a foreign country. Later I read in an Alzheimer's book that families often first realize that something is wrong when they are in an unfamiliar place.

The day I knew for sure something was terribly wrong, we were in our hotel room in the jungle near Palenque. I lay in my underpants on the blue bedspread in the humid, sticky afternoon air, and Julian asked me where his wallet was.

"It's under the green pack," I said, glancing in the direction of the green backpack which lay conspicuously on the dresser.

Julian looked and looked. He scanned all the surfaces in the room. He looked right at the pack, but didn't see it.

"It's under the green pack," I said again. "The green pack. Under the green pack."

He looked at me as blankly as if I had spoken to him in Chinese. I felt a clammy hand of terror clutch my heart. But I pushed away thoughts of what this might mean. I didn't want to think about it. Something ineffable was wrong.

"Something is terribly wrong with Julian," I confessed to two close women friends after that trip. But it wasn't for six months that we eventually scheduled an appointment with a neurologist. Even then, the word "Alzheimer's" never crossed my mind. Only that something very peculiar was going on. "Insidious," the Alzheimer's pamphlets say. "Alzheimer's has an insidious onset."

It's nearly three years since that Yucatan trip. Now I assume that I carry the keys, read the map, keep the money, the whole shebang. We're safe in La Quinta Park Hotel, which is not in a town. Julian can wander around the hotel complex and not really get lost. If we go to Puerto de la Cruz, we walk arm in arm and I've put a little note with the address of our hotel in his pocket.

Tonight is the fourth night we've been here. Returning from a trip to town, I let Julian lead me to our room. He found the stairs. He descended one flight and turned right. So far so good. Then he walked into 90-B.

"Not quite," I said. He backtracked, passed 89, and walked up to Room 87.

"Over here, Julian. Here's our room," I said, opening the door with my key. "Our room number is 89-B."

What a marvel of accomplishment is the normally functioning brain.

"I Know, Dear Heart, I Know"

The rehearsal for the investiture was on Tuesday morning. Manuel picked up Julian and me at the hotel, along with Russ Reiter, a prominent physiologist from Texas, also receiving an honorary degree. Manuel led us into the auditorium where tomorrow's ceremony would take place.

Above the stage hung a red velvet banner with a gold floral border surrounding the university's crest. Stagehands arranged flags on the left side of the stage. Flags of Spain, the Canaries, and the university, Manuel explained. To the right stood eleven flags with elaborate coats of arms and different colors for the various faculties: medicine, economics, humanities, law. I slipped into a seat in the middle of the auditorium to watch.

On stage a short, stocky man with a black moustache and a red sweater shouted directions. Stagehands pushed blue upholstered chairs with carved wooden arms into a double row on the left of the stage, the chairs in which the four honorary professors would sit. Men and women milled about the stage awaiting instructions.

The man in the red sweater turned out to be the protocol director. Holding a clipboard of papers, he shouted in Spanish while Manuel maneuvered Julian and Russ about the stage, translating the directions into English.

"Sit here," he said, pointing to the high-backed chairs. "Now walk to center stage. Now mount the steps to the high wooden benches. Then go back to the blue chairs."

Manuel showed Russ and Julian how they should bow to the "Rectora Magnifica," the rector of the university, the only woman university president in Spain. They practiced the formal embrace, which they would do upon receiving the ring, the medallion, and the fringed lampshade hat, hugging first to the left, then to the right. Manuel embraced Julian and Julian embraced Russ. Russ laughed, hamming it up and embracing everyone in sight.

In the middle of the explanations, a frail, delicate, white-haired gentleman shuffled down the center aisle on the arm of a young, blond woman. As they climbed the steps to the stage, she counted, *"Uno, dos, tres, cuatro, cinco."* Alberto Sartoris, age ninety-one, a distinquished Italian architect, was also receiving a degree. Professor Sartoris was introduced to the folks on stage, and he smiled sweetly as he shook each person's hand.

The fourth man to receive the *honoris causa* was Professor Gregorio Salvador, a leading authority in the Royal Academy of the Spanish Language. As he had been on the faculty of this university and already understood the ceremony, he would not be attending the rehearsal, Manuel explained.

First I sat on a carved wooden bench. Then I moved closer and sat on a blue velvet bench; finally, as no one else was in the audience and as no one seemed to care, I moved right up to the front row and sat on a red velvet, high-backed chair directly below the stage. I lay my hands on the red velvet armrests, crossed my legs, and settled down to watch.

The protocol director seemed harried. He repeated directions to Alberto Sartoris, who practiced the bow to the Rectora Magnifica and the embraces. From the front row I could hear Manuel's explanations of what was happening.

"You go to the right of the stage to be presented with your medallion," he told Russ and Julian. "Then go over here to receive your ring. You'll receive the leather gloves after the ring."

Julian stood quietly and smiled, listening politely as Manuel led him to different positions on the stage. Alberto Sartoris was led around by the blond woman and Russ by a bearded professor from the medical school.

Each honorary professor had his "patron," the sponsor who had recommended him for the degree and who was responsible for him during the ritual. Eventually the patrons would deliver their charges to the Rectora Magnifica, who would place the yellow, fringed hat upon their head, the final act bestowing upon them the degree of *honoris causa.*

The patrons would each make a speech praising the honoree and describing his accomplishments, followed by acceptance speeches. Manuel would deliver Julian's acceptance speech in addition to his introduction.

The ceremony would end when the four new professors, wearing their medallions, rings, and hats, marched to the Rectora Magnifica, alone, without their patrons, laid their hands on a Bible, and read the Latin oath, vowing to honor and defend the University de la Laguna.

Different parts of the ceremony were practiced, but not in order. The Italian professor shuffled about the stage looking confused. Julian sat quietly and smiled, equally bewildered. Russ tried for a while to comprehend it but, as different acts were rehearsed in a seemingly random sequence, he soon gave up.

"I don't understand a thing," he whispered to me from the stage.

"Don't worry," Manuel said. "Your patron will lead you around. All you'll have to do by yourselves is read the Latin oath. And then you'll be reading together."

Suddenly music blared over the loudspeaker, first a few bars of Wagnerian marches, then some measures of "Gaudeamus Igitur," then part of the Star Spangled Banner. Tears suddenly filled my eyes. The music pushed my emotions to the surface, and all the layers of meaning of this event swirled within me.

I sprang from my seat and stood at attention. Russ stood up too. After the U.S. anthem came two more patriotic pieces, the Italian national anthem and the Spanish, Manuel explained.

Waves of pride swelled as I watched Julian up on the stage. Julian had worked hard over thirty years. Last week in Palo Alto, facing the closing of his lab and the loss of his driver's license, he had felt incompetent and insignificant; now suddenly he felt appreciated. My joy intensified thinking of Julian—unable to find his hotel room, remember his birthdate, or even know what town he was in—being so honored. Here was Manuel, about to deliver a fifteen-minute speech praising Julian's accomplishments, and Julian couldn't remember what his work was.

The night before, Manuel had given us a tan book containing a full-page color photograph of the four honorees, followed by their professional biography; in Julian's case, written by Erla, Julian's research associate these past twenty-five years. It also contained each man's bibliography. Julian and I looked over his bibliography that night in bed, scanning his 183 published research papers, beginning in 1960, the year we married.

"You know," Julian confessed sheepishly. "I don't know what any of this work is about."

"I know, dear heart, I know," I had said.

I watched Russ cavorting around on stage, enjoying himself thoroughly, practicing the embraces and waving to an imagined crowd. A man of Julian's age, he would return to his active lab and resume his high-powered career, still going full-steam ahead, a competent, bright, creative man enjoying his prime.

As patriotic music blared from the loudspeakers, the protocol director shouted to lower the volume. He laughed, trying to coordinate the correct music with the actions on stage. Manuel joked and smiled, maneuvered Julian around, and jotted down notes. Julian and Russ danced a little jig to some lively, jolly music we later learned was the Italian national anthem, but Alberto Sartoris smiled and didn't seem to mind.

The rehearsal was going well. The protocol director laughed, Manuel stopped taking notes, the flags stood firmly in place, and Alberto Sartoris and his blond patron approached the edge of the stage.

"*Uno, dos, tres, cuatro, cinco,*" she said again as they stepped down each stair. The folks on stage stood around and chatted. The protocol director looked satisfied. The rehearsal seemed over.

I waved to Julian and winked. I saluted Russ and Manuel. I laughed and cried and wiped my eyes and loved the investiture ceremony already. Then Manuel brought Julian and Russ down the steps and led us all up the auditorium's center aisle.

"We have a one o'clock appointment to meet the Rectora in her office," Manuel said. When Julian disappeared into the men's room, I took Manuel aside.

"But Manuel, Julian won't remember any of what's been practiced," I said. "He won't remember when he's supposed to do what. And besides, you didn't even rehearse things in the right order."

"It's okay," Manuel reassured me. "Russ will go first at each part of the ceremony, and I'll be right by Julian's side except at the very end. As for the Latin oath, it turns out the Spanish professor will read it and all Julian has to say is '*Ego* Doctor Julian Mordecai Davidson.'"

"*Ego* Doctor Julian Mordecai Davidson," Manuel repeated when Julian returned. "That's all you have to say." He whisked us off to meet the Rectora Magnifica in her office. Then he drove us back to the hotel to greet our sons, who had just flown in for tomorrow's ceremony.

"*Ego* Doctor Julian Mordecai Davidson," Manuel had written down on a piece of paper for Julian. Julian kept it in his left shirt pocket. He took out the scrap of paper and read it over and over all that afternoon. As we rested by the pool and hung around with Ben and Jeff at the hotel, I would catch Julian reading the paper quietly to himself.

"*Ego* Doctor Julian Mordecai Davidson." I would whisper to him as we lay on the white plastic lounge chairs by the turquoise pool. "*Ego* Doctor Julian Mordecai Davidson." repeated Ben and Jeff as we ate our lunch of bread, cheese and oranges on our balcony with pink geraniums in a window box and a view of the deep blue sea and the tiny white buildings of Puerto de la Cruz down the coast.

In bed that night, Julian confessed,"You know. It's five things. But I can't do it without reading."

"Try." I modeled it for him. "*Ego* Doctor Julian Mordecai Davidson."

"Doctor . . ." he began.

"*Ego*," I said. "*Ego* Doctor . . ."

"*Ego* Doctor . . . Julian Davidson . . . Mordecai," he said.

"Just say '*ego* Doctor' and your name — Julian Mordecai Davidson."

"*Ego* doctor . . . Julian Davidson . . . Mordecai."

"Julian Mordecai Davidson," I said. "Julian Mordecai Davidson."

"Julian Mordecai Davidson Doctor," he said.

Try as he might, Julian simply could not insert his middle name between his first and last. Trying to remember "Mordecai" threw him completely. The fifth item was just too much.

"Forget the 'Mordecai,'" I said. "*Ego* Doctor Julian Davidson."

"*Ego* Doctor Julian Davidson . . ." I heard across the darkness.

"Terrific," I said. "Good night, my darling, I'm so proud of you." And "*Ego* Doctor Julian Mordecai Davidson" echoed in my dreams all night.

An Unforgettable Day

The phone rang at seven-thirty Wednesday morning, the day of the ceremony. Russ called to wake us up. We showered and dressed in clothes laid out carefully the night before. Julian put on the new black trousers, socks, and shoes requested by Manuel. He wore his new sport jacket and a red tie. I wore a blue paisley dress bought for this occasion after a desperate search through my closet produced nothing appropriate.

Ben and Jeff were tying their ties in the bathroom when I called them for breakfast. Beyond the backs of their starched white shirts, I saw their reflections in the mirror . . . the same height, the same light brown hair, Ben's cut close to his scalp, Jeff's standing up stiff with gel. They slipped on dark jackets and turned to face me. How elegant my two sons looked. I had never before seen either of them in a suit.

The four of us trooped into the hotel dining room, an over-dressed quartet among the other guests wearing colorful shorts and sandals, ready to soak up Canary Island sun. Ben and Jeff grimaced as I snapped photos of my trio around the table, conspicuous enough without my camera's flash.

Promptly at nine Manuel arrived at the hotel to drive us to the university. We climbed the stone steps and entered a large reception area where men in dark suits and women in dressy outfits were assembling.

"Come help Julian dress," Manuel said, leading us into a wood-paneled room off the foyer. There, on plush armchairs, lay the black academic gowns sewn especially for this occasion, according to the measurements I had faxed to Manuel. I had never suspected they were actually sewing Julian a gown. In Stanford academic processions, professors simply borrow gowns from the bookstore.

While Julian, Russ, and Manuel struggled into tuxedo shirts and bow ties, I snipped white threads that held the pleats of the gowns. I fastened Julian's cuff links and clipped on his bow tie, as other wives adjusted their husbands' satin hoods: yellow for medicine, blue for humanities, red for law. I fussed over Russ's hood too, as his wife was in Texas. More black-robed professors filled the room, wearing fringed lampshade hats that matched their satin hoods and wide lace cuffs.

Just before eleven the guests left for the auditorium. Ben, Jeff, Manuel's wife, Maria, and I were escorted to seats of honor on light blue velvet benches in the third row. In front of us were two rows of red velvet high-backed chairs.

Suddenly a trumpet fanfare quieted the room. Through double carved doors marched two young guards in maroon velvet suits trimmed in gold, bearing elaborately carved silver scepters. Behind them marched the black-gowned academicians, first professors in light blue hoods, then red, and last yellow, for medicine, newest of the disciplines.

Heads turned to watch the procession troop down the aisle to take their seats on the red velvet chairs in front of us. There was Manuel, in his yellow mantle and lampshade hat, a head taller than everyone around him. Beside him walked Julian, wearing his black robe and yellow mantle, but hatless, as the four honorary doctors would receive their hats at the ceremony's climax. Behind Julian walked Russ and his sponsor.

Cameras flashed and clicked. Julian looked solemn and dignified. Manuel slipped easily into this pompous role, even though as a radical young professor he had previously scoffed at formal ceremonies, as had Julian over the decades, until his recent awareness that his academic game was nearly over. Why, when we're about to lose something, do we suddenly appreciate it most?

Up the five steps marched the Rectora Magnifica in her black satin hood to sit in the center of the high wooden dais, followed by dignitaries who sat beside her. The four honorees bowed to the Rectora at the top of the steps and then sat down on blue velvet chairs to her right with their sponsors behind them. Manuel escorted Julian, his hand on Julian's arm.

Julian sat straight, head held high, playing the part perfectly. He looked rather like a Jewish pope in a high Catholic mass. So far so good.

The ceremony began with greetings by the Rectora Magnifica. Then each sponsor gave a long speech in Spanish praising the accomplishments of his honoree. Manuel, handsome in his yellow hat, stood at the podium recounting Julian's achievements. I recognized familiar words even in Spanish—*fisiología, endocrinología, testosterone, hypothalamus*. I glanced over at Ben's and Jeff's faces, listening attentively to Manuel. Julian, looking wise and serious, also focused on Manuel, appearing as if he understood Spanish.

Then, one by one—Russ first, Julian second, Alberto Sartoris third, and Gregorio Salvador last—each honoree stepped forward to have a gold ring slipped on his finger, a medallion placed around his neck, white leather gloves presented to him, and, finally, the fringed lampshade hat placed solemnly on his head by the Rectora Magnifica. With each action the music changed, and there were handshakes, the rehearsed double embraces, and the flash of cameras as photographers crouched beneath the stage snapping photos.

If someone went to the wrong place at the wrong time, no one seemed to care. At one point Russ walked to the Rectora Magnifica instead of to the podium to give his speech, but it didn't matter.

After the *doctoris honoris causis* were bestowed with their new titles and hats, each stepped to the podium to deliver his acceptance speech. First Russ spoke in English with a Spanish translation placed on each seat. Then Manuel read Julian's speech, supposedly because Julian had broken his reading glasses.

"Oh, no," I whispered to Maria as Manuel stepped to the

podium to read. "We forgot to remove Julian's glasses as we'd planned."

There was Manuel explaining that he was reading Julian's speech because Julian had broken his glasses, but Julian was wearing his glasses. Oh well, what difference did that make really? It was fine. All my worries had been for naught. How often it is this way.

I watched the faces of the professors on stage as Manuel read Julian's speech. They seemed interested, I imagined. At one point everyone laughed, the first laughter in this solemn ceremony. I knew it was in response to a remark on the effects of castration on the aggressive behavior of Spanish bulls. I promised myself to remember to tell Julian's friend Ben Sachs, who had written the acceptance speech for him, that his joke was successful.

Pride mixed with sadness, appreciation of Julian was tinged with grief that he was being lauded in this two-and-a-half-hour ceremony while unable to write or read his own speech. But the speech was hardly the issue. Mostly I was filled with undiluted joy that Julian was being honored, that he was being fussed over at this precarious time in his life. I felt happy that Ben and Jeff were here to share in this tribute to their father and to learn of his accomplishments about which they were barely aware. I, too, hadn't realized exactly what Julian's contribution to behavioral endocrinology had been. It took this investiture ceremony on Tenerife and Manuel's speech to reveal this part of Julian to his sons and me.

After the last speech the four new honorary doctors crowded around a large Bible in front of the Rectora Magnifica as Professor Salvador read the Latin oath. I waited anxiously for Julian to say his well-rehearsed line. But, as with so many things I fret about, the reading of the oath flashed by without problems. The professors mumbled their names quietly up on the stage, this part of the ceremony over in an instant.

When the three national anthems sounded, the entire audience rose to their feet. During the lively Italian anthem, Julian wagged his head from side to side, in time to the beat. Manuel told us later he was afraid Julian's hat would fall off and roll across the stage.

Then from the balcony came the strains of "Gaudeamus Igitur" sung by a student chorus, followed by the Rectora Magnifica leading the procession down from the stage, along the center aisle, and out into the foyer. There, gowned professors and guests mingled and talked, a melee of colors and Spanish voices.

Ben, Jeff, Maria, and I pushed through the crowd to find Julian and Manuel. Maria took photos standing on the wide stone steps—Manuel with his arm around Julian, Julian hugging me, and the Rectora Magnifica standing between Julian and Manuel. Introductions and congratulations flew around us. Julian beamed and my sons stood close to their dad; I threw my arms around Julian's yellow mantle and squeezed him tight.

Then, my face squashing into the smooth satin of Manuel's hood, I hugged him and stood on tiptoes to kiss his bearded cheek.

"Thank you, Manuel," I said, "for giving us this unforgettable day."

The Coach Becomes a Pumpkin

Two days after we arrived home from Spain, we were back in a speech therapy session at the Veteran's Hospital. The spouses were invited to sit in and observe.

The speech pathologist, Kelly, greeted Julian warmly. "Welcome back," she said. "How was your trip? Tell us about it."

Julian grinned and attempted to say a few sentences about the ceremony and his adventure. He stumbled and fumbled and produced long, vague circumlocutions. It was impossible to understand what he was talking about if you didn't already know.

Kelly listened intently, smiled, and helped Julian out. She filled in missing words and asked him questions to clarify his incomprehensible account, like helping a kindergartner tell about his summer vacation at "show-and-tell."

Julian had brought his new medallion and his gold ring. It was easier for him to speak when he held a concrete object to cue his memory. The medallion and ring were passed around, and the group exclaimed over them. Then Kelly handed out papers listing twenty categories: states on the East Coast, streets near your house, holidays, countries in Europe.

Everyone was to call out words that fit into each category. Long silences preceded any response. I intentionally kept quiet. The husband of a woman with Alzheimer's started offering words. Slowly the Alzheimer's patients caught on and began producing a word or two.

Julian was quiet. He held the paper in his hands and kept his eyes focused on it, clearly embarrassed at being unable to respond. Out of twenty categories, all he produced was "Scotland" when we named countries in Europe.

Next, Kelly shifted to the second activity: a game where we described an object for the others to guess. Description is an important strategy for word-finding difficulties, a problem shared by most people with Alzheimer's, she said.

We were handed a scrap of paper on which was printed a single word: "fork," "harmonica," "mustard," "butterfly," "barbecue," "muffin." Each person in turn would give hints or cues until the word was guessed. I went first, describing my word, "barbecue," until someone figured it out. Julian made no attempt at guessing. Everyone laughed, joked, and made wisecracks. Kelly smiled and gave encouraging remarks, accepting and modifying even incorrect, far-off responses. Julian stayed quiet.

When it was his turn and Kelly handed him his paper, he looked flustered and picked up the first large sheet listing categories. He was having trouble shifting from the first activity to the second.

"What's perseveration?" a friend once asked me when I had told her Julian perseverates a lot.

"It's the difficulty shifting from one task to another," I had told her. I see this often now in Julian's speech. He cannot talk about more than one thing at a time. If we're discussing what we're doing tonight, I can't also mention what's happening tomorrow. I can explain only one thing. If he has a dentist appointment at two, a doctor appointment at four, and we're having coffee in between, that's more than he can handle.

Words from a topic previously discussed insert themselves into later sentences. If I know what we've been talking about the past hour and what things are currently on Julian's mind, then I can sometimes make sense out of his word substitutions and sort them out. There's often some fascinating, connecting link between the inappropriate word he's used and a previous conversation or something I know he's thinking about. Or between the word used and the word intended according to sound—"Spain" for "rain," "deter" for "deteriorated," "keefa" for "coffee." How fascinating this might be if it weren't my husband.

"Julian," Kelly said. "Look at the word on the paper."

Julian looked frantically back and forth from the large paper to the small.

"Look at the little paper," she said, pointing to it. Julian had a hard time looking where she pointed.

I had noticed this difficulty in his ability to look where I pointed all last week. In the hotel on Tenerife, he couldn't focus when I pointed to the sign showing the room numbers. He took a long time locating what I pointed out to him: "See those black volcanic rocks. See that green parrot. See that beautiful carved wooden balcony." He would scan around before he found it.

Julian picked up his bit of paper and read his word silently. But he didn't give any hints. Kelly prompted him, cued him and urged him on with leading questions.

Finally he said, "Eat, something you eat . . ."

"Eat?" Kelly said. "You eat this? You don't eat these," she said. Then she said, "Oh, I see. It's part of the word you're looking at. Look at the whole word."

"Go up," Julian said. "High . . . go up high . . . in the air."

I began asking questions, like the games we used to play on car trips with the children. And finally the group correctly guessed his word: "butterfly."

But after that, Julian hung his head and was embarrassed.

He didn't take another turn and he didn't attempt to guess anyone else's word.

I felt near tears, though I tried to continue participating cheerfully. These were the same activities I had used with my brain-injured, language-impaired seven-year-olds at the Children's Health Council. And Julian was less able to do these tasks than some of them. Here was "Excelentisimo Señor," "Doctor Honoris Causa," the man who had looked so wise and dignified in his academic gown exactly one week earlier. The man whose work Manuel had praised for fifteen minutes in his speech, the man who had been honored and toasted. It broke my heart.

A year ago Helen, the psychiatric nurse at the VA Alzheimer's and Memory Disorder Clinic, asked me if I would like to get involved with the speech pathologist researching the literature on Alzheimer's and language and perhaps help with some experimental therapy groups. I never responded and now I understand why. It's too painful. I used to be fascinated by the academic, intellectual topic of language and the brain. But now it's Julian, my darling Julian, whose brain is slowly dying and with whom I long to speak.

I swallowed these thoughts and took my next turn. "Mustard" was my word. I made funny comments, cracked jokes, and responded to the others. Still Julian remained silent.

When Kelly announced the hour was up, Julian said, "Can I say something?"

"Of course."

"It's worse in here," he said. "I feel so bad. I know it's to help us, but I feel terrible. I can't think of any words. My mind goes blank."

Julian has explained to me how difficult he finds these speech sessions. He goes because he hopes they may help him, but he doesn't enjoy them. I remembered when I was a speech therapist how hard it was for the children to work directly in their area of weakness. I had tried to explain this to Julian on many days when he left the VA feeling discouraged.

"It is hard," Kelly said. "But these exercises can help you

when you can't think of a word." Then she asked each member of the group how they felt about the sessions. Julian's face relaxed and I saw he was relieved to have participated by bringing up something of use.

I remembered Julian last week sitting on the stage in Tenerife, wearing his black gown and yellow hat, his white gloves and medallion. I heard again the medieval chorus singing "Gaudeamus Igitur." I looked around the table at Julian and the other Alzheimer's patients and their spouses in the speech therapy session at the VA. Our royal coach has turned back into a pumpkin.

Letting Go

Directly after the speech therapy session at the VA, Julian and I walked over to Building 4 for the New Couples' Group. Ten chairs were set in a circle in the conference room of the Alzheimer's and Memory Disorder Clinic. The past few times, several couples had come, but this time only Julian and I showed up.

Helen greeted us and we pulled three chairs close together, our knees almost touching.

"So, how was your trip?" Helen's dark eyes looked directly at Julian.

Helen listened intently to Julian's rambling account of our Canary Islands adventure. I bit my tongue and let him speak. I didn't interrupt, fill in missing words, clarify vague circumlocutions or retell anecdotes. It's hard for me to button up my urge to speak for him, but I did.

All I said was, "It was like a fairy story . . . like Cinderella going to the ball. And now we're home." Did I mean Julian was like Cinderella? Or me? Curiously, I think I meant both.

"The trip sounds wonderful," Helen said. "I'm glad it went well."

"I want to thank you," I said, "for your advice."

We did what Helen said: half of what we would ordinarily

have done. We left twice the time we usually allowed for transitions. We rested and hung around the hotel.

"Julian let me carry the tickets, passports, and money and didn't argue about it. He didn't dash off in airports or plazas to look at things, like he did last year. It made the trip easier," I said.

"Yes," Helen said in her soft, calm voice. "All that helps. Leave plenty of time. Don't rush. Avoid fatigue and hurried transitions. Go slow. You need more time for everything."

"As long as we have you to ourselves," I said, "I would like to talk about something else. Julian still has a hard time giving up the car."

I told Helen how after we returned from the Canaries, I removed the car key from his key ring.

"I didn't tell him. I just took it off. He was furious when he found out. He shook his finger at me and shouted, 'You're in trouble! You're in real trouble! It's my car!' He stormed off and was mad all day."

"Maybe I should have told him beforehand?"

Helen turned to Julian. In her calm voice she said, "It's hard, Julian, to let go of the car. But try not to fight over it. Try to just let it go.

"Ann isn't doing this to you," Helen added. "She isn't restricting you. You'll have more freedom if you let certain things go."

Helen explained how in ten years of working with Alzheimer's patients, she'd seen two types.

"Some people let go of areas where they're likely to have trouble," she said. "They plan around their limitations and have more freedom and activity in the long run. Others deny difficulties. They refuse to believe they have a problem and they get into trouble in a catastrophic way—getting lost for days, having an accident, or hurting themselves. Then they get limited even further."

I kept quiet and listened. Julian listened, too, seeming to take in her words. So much better for Helen to tell him than me.

"It's not just driving," Helen continued. "If you can realize that your judgment isn't always accurate, you'll be better off. You'll have more freedom. Learn to trust those who love you. Trust Ann to tell you what's safe. She's not trying to control you. She has your best interests at heart."

I buttoned my lip and prayed he heard her. Julian looked sober, his blue eyes staring at Helen as she talked.

Then Julian shifted the topic to his pending "retirement." In a month his lab will fold up. His staff will leave. His office is being dismantled. For the first time in his adult life, Julian will have no place to go and no structure to his days.

I'm glad he brought this up. It preoccupies him. He's terribly anxious.

"Retirement is a huge change in everyone's life," I said. "But harder for Julian. Work has been his main activity. He can't do what he had always planned to do when retired: write. And work with Amnesty International or a Middle East peace group."

"Are *you* worried about where Julian will go?" Helen asked me.

Suddenly I realized my anxiety was as high as Julian's. How would life be when he no longer went off to work each morning and returned home each night? When weekdays and weekends took on the same rhythm? When he was around all the time? Of course I'm worried.

"Things will evolve," I said. "He can increase his time at the Food Closet. Continue going to his faculty study in the library each morning." For a while longer, anyway, I thought to myself.

"We'll find some classes he could take." I also had secret hopes he might get interested in gardening, cooking, or helping more around the house—nonverbal tasks. Maybe he could do housework in a relaxed, enjoyable, Zen sort of way.

"Before enlightenment—hew wood, carry water," he always told me and I remind him now. "After enlightenment—hew wood, carry water."

Maybe he could learn to wash dishes the way Thich Nhat Hanh describes. Maybe I could learn to do *my* ever-increasing chores in a more calm, accepting manner?

Helen pushed her dark, shoulder-length hair back from her forehead, looked at both of us, and smiled. I looked at my watch. The hour was up.

"Thank you, Helen," I said. "We had you all to ourselves today. We were lucky indeed."

Julian and I walked out to the car together, arm in arm. I felt calm and relaxed as I slid into the driver's seat and Julian got in the passenger side. And it was slowly feeling natural that way.

Winter 1992–93

We held each other close in the dark.

Two Locks, Two Bikes

I stretched out my arms from under the blankets and opened my eyes. My bare legs felt warm between the sheets. December morning sun slanted in through half-drawn drapes, making a puddle of sunlight on the carpet.

Julian stood beside the bed, wearing his maroon pajama bottoms and buttoning his shirt.

"Hi, sweetie," I said.

"I want . . . today . . . you know . . . that place where I . . . you know . . . it's free . . . and I go there . . . and I haven't . . ."

"You mean the Palo Alto Clinic? You want your blood test today?"

Periodically Julian gets his blood drawn for a cholesterol check. For years he's gone early in the morning on his bike before eating breakfast. We'd planned last night for me to take him today.

"I'll take you in the car," I reminded him. "And we'll go out to breakfast afterwards. How's that?"

Julian has one bike at home, so he could have ridden there. But his second bike was at Stanford, locked outside the library, where it had been for nearly a week. We had had another bike fiasco two days earlier. The day before yesterday, Julian had limped home, red faced and sweaty, at seven P.M. when I had expected him at five.

He stomped through the kitchen door, his mouth set in a grim line. He said nothing and headed off to the bedroom.

"Terrible day. Terrible day," he muttered.

"Did you lose your bike?" I guessed, as he had obviously walked home. His brown bike had been missing for five days. He had ridden his white bike this morning and that was now obviously lost too.

"No . . . yes . . . it's . . . I don't know . . . it's not there . . . I don't know what happened . . ." His eyes were downcast and he wouldn't look at me. He sounded the way he had in October when he lost the Toyota.

"It's okay, Julian. We'll go back to Stanford and find your bike," I said. "Let's go right now." In the car driving to the library, where I knew he had been, I quizzed him slowly and gently.

"Were you in the library all day? Did you go somewhere for lunch?"

Parking the car near the library where his faculty study is located, we scanned the nearly empty bike racks which surrounded the building. Searching for a bike during winter break was easy. The gray metal bars held only a few bikes scattered here and there, so different from the hundreds of bikes which fill the racks when Stanford is in session.

Immediately I spied his brown bike, locked, mercifully, to the bike rack. "Voilà!" I said, feeling encouraged. "So far so good."

But Julian had no key to unlock it. He didn't have his regular key chain, nor did he have the key to the bike lock.

"All we have to do is find the key to unlock the brown bike. We'll look at home tonight. Now we'll search for the white bike. Did you eat lunch at Stanford today?" I asked. "Did you buy a sandwich?"

With Julian plodding behind me, I headed straight for the nearby Education Building, where I knew they sold food. There, right outside the door, stood his white bike. The bike cable was looped through the spokes of both wheels, the two ends carefully placed one atop the other, but no lock linked them together.

"We're in luck today," I said as Julian wheeled his white bike to the car. Back home, I felt triumphant seeing the white bike back in its usual place in our courtyard.

So this morning, when I offered to drive Julian to the clinic for his blood test, I had an ulterior motive: to drive him to the Stanford library afterward so he could then come home on his brown bike.

"Julian, get the key for your brown bike," I said this morning.

He looked at me blankly.

"The brown bike, the brown bike," I repeated. "Please find the key for the brown bike lock."

"They let me in . . . they always let me in . . . I don't need a key . . . the nice man . . ."

"No," I said, jumping out of bed and slipping on my jeans, turtleneck, and sneakers. "The bike key. The key to the lock for the brown bike."

"I can always get in the library," he said.

"Julian. You're talking about the library. I'm talking about the brown bike. Your brown bike."

"I'll take my bike," he said, putting on his shoes.

"Julian, remember, we found your brown bike. Remember, it was locked. If you get the key, you can bring the brown bike home."

Every time I mentioned the brown bike, he responded thinking of the library. I couldn't get through to him. My voice got shriller.

"The brown bike! The brown bike!" I yelled.

"Stop shouting at me! You ruin everything." His tight-set lips arched sadly downward. I knew he couldn't help the way he was, but I couldn't stop feeling agitated. My chest felt tight. My forehead taut. My voice constricted. All the delicious feelings I had had upon awakening were gone. I had only been awake ten minutes.

I waved my hand as if erasing a blackboard. "Scratch that," I said gently, but the gentleness seemed forced. It wasn't genuine. Julian knew it too. "Let's start again."

But before I knew what was happening, we were back at it, each of us caught in an endless loop. I kept trying to explain about the brown bike and lost key. He kept talking about the library. As we got in the car to drive to the clinic, I muttered to myself, "I'm going crazy."

I knew I wasn't, but it felt that way. I drove to the clinic with Julian sitting sullenly beside me. "Why do you ruin everything?" he said.

Maybe my patience ran thin because I had planned to prepare the overdue taxes this morning, a task I'm tense about. I had thought I had a month to get the papers ready, but I learned last night the accountant wanted them two days ago. Maybe it was because I had watched a video yesterday on Alzheimer's borrowed from the public library, a depressing series of vignettes showing Alzheimer's patients in varying stages of decline. The video was entitled *You Are Not Alone,* the exact opposite of how I felt.

In the car, I flicked on the radio to listen to the news. Julian pushed the button off. I shoved in a tape and Vivaldi blared from the speakers. Julian pushed that off too.

"You should have married Mother Teresa," I snapped. We drove to the clinic in silence.

While Julian was getting his blood test in the lab, I flipped through a *National Geographic,* looking at photographs of Tanzania, Egypt, and Mauritius and wishing I were there.

When Julian returned to the waiting room with a Band-Aid in the crook of his left elbow, I took his arm. "Let's go have breakfast," I said as we zipped up our jackets. "Good Earth or Peninsula Creamery?"

He didn't answer. "Let's walk." I slipped my arm along his. We walked in silence down cold sidewalks strewn with mushy, brown leaves to the coffee shop where I know he likes to eat after his blood tests.

In the Creamery, we slid into a smooth, maroon vinyl booth. Overhead fans circulated warm air. Plastic Christmas greens were looped along the walls, held by lit-up Santa faces. On the Formica table, jars of mustard, catsup, and Heinz steak sauce supported menus in plastic folders. We loved this old coffee shop, straight out of the fifties.

Over my scrambled eggs, toast, and hash browns and his Belgian waffle, we began chatting about when he was a boy in Glasgow, a safe, familiar topic. Full sentences returned. He gave me a quarter of his waffle. I gave him most of my hash browns. I poured a lot of syrup on the waffle and ate all my toast. We drank three refills of watery coffee.

En route back to the car we stopped at a Jewish bookstore and an art store to have a print of Glasgow University framed.

Then I drove Julian to the library. We parked the car and walked toward the bike racks. "Here's your brown bike," I said quietly. "If you have the key, you can ride it home."

He pulled from his pocket a square metal lock with a key protruding from it.

"No, Julian. That's the lock and key for your *white* bike." I vowed to immediately buy a new lock with two keys and I would keep one. If he couldn't find the key, I planned to borrow a wire cutter and cut the old lock. It was now eleven-fifteen and I hadn't yet started the taxes.

But, lo and behold, he suddenly produced from his briefcase a small silver key on a red plastic tag. He slipped the key in the lock and it snapped open. Hallelujah!

I hugged Julian, smiled, and watched him head into the library. Then I drove home to prepare the taxes for our accountant. Two bikes. Two locks. Both keys. Life this morning returned to normal. Today was looking good.

All My Hopes

Each Sunday I have a phone conversation with Magda, my oldest friend. Either she calls me, or I call her in Los Angeles. Now that she's over eighty, I treasure these calls, cherishing her voice and wisdom.

"And how is Ann?" she asks in her Hungarian accent after we've chatted awhile about this and that, about my grandchildren and hers, our trip to the beach, her grandson's wedding.

"What's going on? How are you—really?"

She's one of the few people I know who truly asks and is prepared to listen. I can say anything, whatever's on my mind. Only with Magda do I say what I feel and know I will be heard. Some therapists may listen this way, too, hard and nonjudgmentally, only you pay them to hear you. And your time is up after fifty minutes.

As we speak I clutch my portable phone with one hand while the other unloads the dishwasher, fills it again with dirty dishes, tidies the kitchen, and scours the sink.

"I'm in a kind of holding pattern," I say. "No highs, no lows. No traumas or dramas. Just chugging along.

"But Julian's had a turning point," I tell her. "At the Alzheimer's couples' group, the psychiatric nurse leading the group was very frank with him. Julian asked directly, 'Is this disease progressive?' And she answered clearly, 'Yes. It is progressive.' He really heard it, let the words in and glimpsed the implications."

"Terrible," Magda says, "to take away hope."

She tells me they don't do it that way in Hungary. Doctors don't give people a hopeless prognosis or tell them they have a terminal or progressive disease, leaving them with no hope. "That's terrible," she repeats.

"But she said it kindly," I say. "She was concerned and supportive."

The nurse likes Julian, I know. She admires and respects him. A medical researcher herself, she probably identifies with him; Alzheimer's could happen to her.

"Helen said nothing happens suddenly," I add. "You don't wake up one day and suddenly find you can't do something or are incapable."

"Terrible," Magda repeats. "Maybe it won't happen to Julian. Maybe he'll be different. Maybe they'll find a cure. There's new research every day."

A rush of emotion rises in my gut. Is it anger? Feeling misunderstood? Having the threat of Julian's condition minimized? Maybe I *am* wrong?

But I say quietly to Magda, "I don't believe there'll be any cures for Julian. I believe he'll deteriorate and slowly get worse."

"You've got to have hope," Magda protests. As a child, she loved fairy tales about princes, princesses, and fairy godmothers. She loved magic. "Look at all the people with cancer who are given six months to live and are alive five years later."

"But this is Alzheimer's," I say. "I don't have hope for a cure. Though we don't really know what will happen."

"No one ever knows what will happen," she says.

"We all live with uncertainty," I say, thinking of three women in my cancer support group who've already died and three others with incurable recurrences. "No one knows," I say, flashing again on the thought that Magda is over eighty.

"People need hope," she says. "You can't take away hope."

"I agree," I say, "I have plenty of hopes: I hope Julian will remain as well as he is for a long time to come. I hope he'll finish his autobiography and he'll be happy. I hope I'll learn to live with his illness without destroying my own life. I hope I can live with joy and good cheer much of the time. I hope I'll be able to handle what needs to be done. I hope my friends won't abandon me as Julian gets worse."

"Here's one who won't," Magda interrupts my list and states emphatically.

"I hope I'll stay well so I can care for him. I hope I'll have a long and healthy life. I hope we'll have more good years together. I hope I'll be able to manage. I hope I can accept my burdens and deal joyfully with whatever comes. I hope I can remain loving throughout this ordeal. I hope we'll have good times over Christmas vacation when all the kids come home," I tell Magda. "These are some of my hopes."

"Dear Ann," she says. "My dearest Ann."

In Candy Land

"Gramma, Gramma, let's play." Three-year-old Celina ran into the kitchen carrying the flat white box. "Let's play Candy Land."

I was washing the dishes before dressing for the Christmas open house Julian and I had been invited to. Karen and the children were spending the weekend, and they would stay home while we went to the party. Julian eagerly anticipated this annual event held for professors at the university president's house.

"I want to go," Julian said as soon as the invitation came. "When do we go to that big guy's house?" he had asked nearly every day for the past month.

"Let's play Candy Land," Celina urged.

There was time for a quick game, I thought. "Go get Grampa and Antar and Mommy," I said. "Tell them to come play."

Celina sat cross-legged on the family room carpet and opened the folded board. She grabbed a red plastic gingerbread man. "I'm red," she announced as the others settled themselves on the floor around the game. "You be green," she said to her older brother, who plopped beside her. "You're yellow, Grampa! And Mommy's blue."

Antar arranged the small white cards into a neat stack, and we began.

"Double green," Antar said, moving his man to the second green square along the curving path leading to Candy Castle. "Orange." Celina competantly advanced her man to the orange square. "Double purple," Karen announced.

Julian sat cross-legged on the floor on his side of the board, watching the children begin the game.

"Your turn, Grampa," Antar said. "Take a card."

Julian looked blank and smiled at Antar.

"Here, Grampa. Here's your card." Antar handed Julian a card from the stack. "What color is it, Grampa?" Antar asked, in the intonation pattern of his second-grade teacher.

"Green," said Julian.

"Put your man here, Grampa." Antar pointed to the appropriate green square. Julian looked at the stack of cards. "*Here*, Grampa." Then Julian looked at Karen, unable to focus where Antar pointed. I moved Julian's man to the green square.

"Grandpa and I will be a team," I said. "We'll play together."

"Double blue," shouted Celina, marching her man to the second blue square, past Peppermint Forest and Gumdrop Pass.

Julian began talking about the Christmas party in a vague rambling way, but Karen ignored him and made some comment about the game. Julian's mouth drooped after she cut him off. He grew silent and looked away.

"Mommy," Antar said. "You shouldn't interrupt Grampa when he's talking."

Karen looked thoughtfully at Antar, nodded, then turned to Julian. "What did you say, Dad?" she asked. "What about the party?"

The game continued. For half an hour Karen, Julian, Antar, Celina, and I played Candy Land, each in turn drawing a card from the top of the stack and moving our plastic gingerbread men along the path of colored squares. Squeals of delight if we drew a double color and advanced forward, or got a lollipop card and moved ahead to that special spot; shrieks of "Oh, no" if we drew a card requiring return to an earlier position.

Despite repeated explanations, Julian never did understand the game. But he sat on the floor with us around the bright board, picking the top card when Antar told him it was his turn and loudly calling out his color. ... "Green." "Red." "Yellow." Then Antar or Celina would move his plastic man to where it should go.

As we played, I began worrying about the party. We were due at the president's house at four. I had hesitated when the invitation came, dreading going with Julian to a cocktail party full of professors. It's a strain to cover for him, embarrassing when he says inappropriate things and there's no chance for me to explain. "But he's worked at Stanford thirty years," I told myself. "Why shouldn't he go to the president's party?"

We showered and dressed. Julian put on his new black trousers and gray tweed sport coat bought especially for the Canary Islands. He knotted his red tie before the mirror; he looked great.

Walking up to the president's mansion, I hesitated, swallowing my nervousness before ringing the bell. A maid in a black dress and white apron opened the door, took my coat, and ushered us into the bright living room filled with well-dressed couples standing with wineglasses in hand, talking and eating. A fire blazed in the huge stone fireplace to my right; a Christmas tree reached from floor to ceiling, covered with tiny twinkling lights. Poinsettias dotted the room in clay pots with red velvet bows. I took Julian's arm and plunged into the crowd, my eyes searching for someone I knew.

Crossing the living room and going outside onto the less crowded terrace, we headed for the food: a long table covered with brass trays of jumbo prawns, stuffed mushrooms, and crab cakes. I found myself standing near a woman I recognized, so I helped myself to a prawn and started to chat. Julian stood quietly beside me, sipping his wine and scanning the table. He hated shrimp and he wouldn't eat crab cakes. No desserts out here on the terrace; knowing Julian's sweet tooth, I knew he was looking for chocolate. Three sips of wine and I stopped worrying about Julian. The prawns were fabulous, huge and juicy, the tangy tomato sauce just right. By now I was in a heated conversation about gay and lesbian youth needing information in high schools, and when I looked up, Julian was gone.

Gazing around the terrace, I couldn't see him. For a moment I felt anxious, but I quickly realized he was safe. He wouldn't leave the house. What could happen, really? Only that he might meet someone he knew who didn't know about his Alzheimer's and they would have a vague, weird, inappropriate conversation, and then they would know. That's the worst that could happen.

And why shouldn't Julian get dressed up in his new clothes, come to the president's party, mix and mingle with his colleagues, and enjoy himself in a festive scene?

I sipped my wine, nibbled crab cakes and tasted little hot quiches that waitresses brought around. A couple I knew came to the table, and we exchanged updates on what our kids were doing. Before long I looked up and saw only a few people left on the terrace. Glancing at my watch, I realized the designated party time was nearly over. An hour and a half had passed. Where was Julian?

Wandering back into the almost empty living room, I saw the dining area at the far end, hidden before by the crowd. A long table stretched across it was filled with sweets: lemon layer cake, marzipan, trays of cookies, a glass bowl of trifle, and two silver platters of huge chocolate truffles, larger than golf balls. At the end of the table stood Julian, a half-eaten truffle in one hand and a green paper plate holding three more truffles in the other. Seeing me, he grinned.

"Hi, darling," I said, wiping a smudge of chocolate from his beard.

"Isn't this great?" he said, looking joyful and relaxed, surrounded by chocolate, here in Candy Land.

The Only Thing to Do Was Laugh

All Christmas Day I didn't feel well. During our festive brunch, the opening of presents, and dinner preparations, my head ached and my throat felt raw. After dinner I couldn't wait to say good night and crawl into bed.

The next morning I slept late, carefree after the Christmas bustle. Ben and Jeff had driven to San Francisco for a few days to see friends. Beiçola was in Brazil visiting his family, and Karen and the children were staying with Julian and me for two weeks. She and Beiçola had decided to remain in their house even though the neighborhood had its problems, but she preferred staying with us while he was away. Great timing. I let myself collapse, knowing my capable daughter was in charge.

When I awoke, my throat felt on fire and my chest felt as if concrete had been poured into it. Karen brought me orange juice and felt my forehead.

"You're really hot, Mom," she said, handing me a thermometer.

"One hundred and two," she announced. "Stay in bed. I'll take care of everything."

I sank into my pillows, unable to express how much I appreciated hearing those words.

That morning I alternately drifted off to sleep, then woke in a sweat. Julian wandered in and out, looking at me as if I should get up. I heard TV cartoons blaring from the family room. Karen appeared from time to time with cups of water and tea with honey.

"Come on, Dad," she said to Julian. "Let Mom sleep. Come help the kids and me make soup." And Karen led Julian out of our room while I slid into a delicious nap.

When I got up to shuffle to the bathroom, I saw them all around the butcher block in the kitchen's center. Antar and Celina sat on two high stools, Antar slicing carrots and Celina breaking string beans. Julian stood next to them, cutting onions.

"Boo hoo," he cried, dramatically wiping his weeping eyes. With each mock cry, Celina laughed.

Later Karen returned to my room to announce she was taking Antar, Celina, and Julian to the library. I fell asleep as soon as they left. When I woke up, Julian and Karen stood by my bed. My breath wheezed in and out of my throat. Karen took my temperature again: 104.

Winter 1992–93

"I don't like the way you look, Mom," Karen said. She called the clinic and the receptionist told her to bring me to Urgent Care. Karen collected everyone's jackets—Antar's, Celina's, mine, and Julian's—and we all piled into her car and drove to the clinic. She took Julian and the kids to a nearby park while I slumped in a blue vinyl chair in the waiting room, the other chairs filled with people coughing and sneezing.

When I was finally taken to an examining room, a young woman doctor, looking no older than Karen, took my temperature and listened through her stethoscope to my chest. "Bronchitis," she said. "I'm writing a prescription for antibiotics. There's a bad flu going around. A week to ten days before you'll feel completely better."

Back home in bed, I lay shivering and sweating. I threw off the covers and drank cold water. Then I huddled under two afghans, shaking. Over the next few days, I slept and dozed and woke and slept again. I couldn't remember ever feeling so sick. Julian tiptoed in and out; often I saw him sitting on the bed looking worried.

Karen appeared with Jell-O and soup, but I could eat nothing. How grateful I felt realizing I could collapse in bed; with Karen here, I didn't have to do anything. Thoughts of one day being seriously ill, maybe with a breast cancer recurrence, crossed my mind. How would I manage if I became sick while Julian needed me?

Lying flat on my back, too weak to get up, I realized that my assumptions about caring for Julian were based on my being healthy and well. I remembered when Julian was first diagnosed with Alzheimer's. Only a year earlier I had been "the patient," just recovering from chemotherapy, feeling vulnerable and dependent on Julian. His diagnosis, though, destroyed forever any possibility that he would care for me.

But I couldn't solve that dilemma now. I just had to trust that somehow I would figure out how to handle whatever eventually needed to be done.

My competent daughter put on her Superwoman cape and flew around: making soup, shopping, playing games with the kids, baking cookies with Julian, taking them all out to the park to play.

Once, when she sat by my bed handing me juice, she said, "I don't know how you do it, Mom. How do you live every day with Dad?" Her lip quivered and her eyes filled with tears. "I didn't realize how he was until I stayed here awhile. Until I spent time alone with him . . ."

I took her cool hand and squeezed it.

"It's so sad, Mom," she said.

"Yes . . . it is." Brushing away my tears, I told her how lucky I was to have her here. Then I described the woman in the Alzheimer's group who had said when she had bronchitis, no friends or family were near enough to help her. She had to get up and cook for her husband while she was sick.

"I appreciate, darling, all you've done."

"But it's you and Dad who've done so much for me. . . ."

My mind flashed back to when Julian helped rescue Karen from an abusive boyfriend, to the time he took her with him to a conference in Mexico City.

Two thumps and Celina's loud cry from the family room interrupted my thoughts, and Karen jumped up to see what happened.

A few days later the time came for Karen to leave. My temperature was back to normal, although my chest still felt full of cement. I wheezed and had trouble breathing, but I felt better. Karen filled the fridge wih Jell-O, black beans, minestrone, and leek and potato soup.

"Sure you'll be okay, Mom?" she asked, zipping her coat. Beiçola was due at the airport in two hours, and she was eager to see him. Ben and Jeff would be back tomorrow.

"I'm here," Julian said. "I'll take care of her."

"Dad's here," I said. "I'll be fine."

After Karen left, a wave of nausea washed through me. "Julian, Julian," I called, lying still, not wanting to move for fear I would throw up. "Bring me a pan. I'm going to be sick."

Moments later Julian appeared, handing me a ballpoint pen. Then, when I asked him to please bring a glass of water, he brought me a saucer and an empty cup. What was there to do but laugh?

I thought of Thich Nhat Hanh and breathed deeply in and out. "I'm okay," I reminded myself. "Right now, I'm really okay." And I got up to get myself a drink of water.

A New Year, a New Life

I drove home from the airport down the dark freeway, alone with Julian, blinking back tears. At midnight I had delivered Jeff and his girlfriend to the departure gate at United Airlines. I had taken Ben to the airport a few days before. A swift hug, a kiss, promises to phone when they arrived—and these sons of mine are gone.

The holidays were crammed with commotion, jolly meals, laughter, and late night videos. The kids and grandchildren came and went. I was over the flu. Now we were back to just the two of us. How would things be now?

Of course, I picked a fight with Julian as we undressed and got into bed. He had turned the heat up too high, I turned it down, and he put it up again. We slept last night back to back, silent, cold, not touching. This morning, the first since all the kids had left, found Julian uncertain what to do.

He hung around forlornly this morning as I dressed for my yoga class. Somehow he ended up coming too. He lay down on a blue mat in the gym at the community center in a room full of women. He tried the movements and postures, only he never quite had the correct leg up or the right arm extended. The yoga teacher bent over him several times, giving him special directions or positioning his body. At one point she came to where I was lying and whispered, "Does he hear all right?"

"Yes," I said. "But he doesn't understand. I'll explain later."

After that she stopped going to Julian to help him assume the postures. She just let him do whatever he could do and didn't correct him. Out of the corner of my eye, I watched him unable to follow her verbal directions or to imitate the movements and poses.

After class, when Julian sat in the corner putting on his tennis shoes, the teacher came to me with a quizzical expression on her face.

"He has trouble following directions," I explained. "He has Alzheimer's."

"Oh, no," she said. "I didn't know." I've known this yoga teacher for years. She looked at me with sorrow in her eyes. "My father has Alzheimer's, too, only he's eighty-five."

"Julian can come anytime," she said quickly. "He's welcome to drop in and do whatever he can."

Tears sprang to my eyes. "I appreciate that," I said, grateful for her kindness.

But I realized that Julian's presence changes the class for me. Yoga would be good for him, yes. We've been talking about him taking yoga "now that he's retired." But *my* yoga class? How did it happen that he came to my yoga class? Five years ago we had taken yoga together and I loved it. I enjoyed doing things with him then and always yearned to spend more time together than he had available. Now he has endless time: my newest challenge. Do I want Julian in my yoga class?

After yoga we drove to Stanford to search for his brown bike, which has been lost again, since last Thursday, somewhere on campus. We walked around two libraries, the student union, and the medical school, scrutinizing hundreds of bicycles chained and locked to gray metal racks. But we couldn't find it.

Then I drove him to the campus bike shop, where I found Keith, the shop owner, who has serviced Julian's bikes for twenty-five years and who has sold him four used bikes in the past six months.

Sometimes I felt crazy looking for lost keys and lost bikes. I had heard the stories about Alzheimer's patients getting lost. But I wanted Julian to be as independent as possible. I decided to let him ride his bike alone to Stanford, as he had done for thirty years, until he showed me he no longer could. I could not restrict him prematurely because "something might happen." At this stage anyway, I would not keep him home like a prisoner. As a consequence we had to keep buying bikes.

"Hi, Keith. We need another one," I said. "A junky three-speed, the cheaper the better." I glanced at the $200 and $300 price tags on the new bicycles.

"Another bike?" Keith looked at me quizzically.

As Julian examined bikes in one section, I took Keith aside.

"My husband has Alzheimer's," I said. "You may have guessed. He forgets his bike lock or key, doesn't lock them, and the bikes get stolen. Or he can't remember where he's parked the bike."

"Oh," said Keith matter-of-factly. "I knew something was wrong. Don't worry. I'll find him a bike. I don't have one here now, but I know his frame size and the kind of handlebars he likes. Call me in a few days."

"Thank you," I said again, appreciative of these random acts of kindness, however small. Empathetic expressions from people, like those of the yoga teacher and Keith, make such a difference.

Leaving the bike shop, I dropped Julian near the student union on campus. "Where are you going now?" I asked. "To the library? To your office?"

He looked at me blankly and got out of the car.

"We'll call Keith in two days about the bike," I said. "You'll have a bike soon. It's sunny and bright today. It won't be bad to walk home. Enjoy the walk. See you tonight, darling." And I drove off, leaving him standing in the road, feeling like I used to feel leaving my kindergartners on the first day of school. How would they manage?

He can't solve the questions of where to go and what to do. I must create a structure. I could call the Jewish Community Center to see if they have classes or lectures he might attend. I could call the Senior Center to inquire about their music appreciation class taught by the teacher of the Yiddish Chorus. Maybe he could spend more time at the Food Closet? If only he would get interested in gardening. Could he take an art class? Or ceramics? How much longer will he be able to get around by himself on his bike, even if he manages not to lose it?

My heart raced, plans swam around in my head. But I no longer felt tentative. I knew exactly what I must do. At home I took out a blank sheet of paper and printed in large capital letters: "JANUARY 19, 1993—TO DO." I started my list—programs to call, classes to check on, brochures to request—and began piecing together a different life for Julian at the start of this special, new year.

"I Hear You," Her Eyes Said

Julian stayed home today. He didn't get dressed. He had nowhere to go, no plans, and no appointments.

Yesterday he had put on his striped office shirt and left the house. He probably went to his faculty study in the library, though I can't imagine what he did there. He can hardly read. He no longer writes meaningful phrases, much less a sentence, yet he stubbornly clings to his thirty-year routine of "going to work." He was gone all day and came home for supper.

But this morning when I went to yoga, I left him wearing pajamas, and he was still in them when I returned. He had cleaned up the kitchen and was sitting in his study next to our bedroom. The red coils of his electric heater glowed cheerily, and his little study was cozy and warm. But he looked so forlorn, even though he greeted me with a hug. He had decided to "work at home," he told me, sorting papers and tidying his desk.

At noon he emerged wearing the long, gray flannel nightshirt Beiçola gave him for Christmas. It hung down over his trousers, and he had put a navy blue sweatshirt over it. He was an odd mixture of dressed and undressed. Just as he is an odd mix of adult and child, wise and simple, the man I love and the man I've lost.

For lunch I dumped Campbell's soup into a saucepan, sliced an apple, and made toast. We sat down at the table together. He needed me, I could tell. Almost everyone else has left his life. He wouldn't speak to anyone today except me. I knew he wanted to chat, but I had phone calls to make, bills to pay, my writing, and volunteer tasks to think about. My oncologist said she would call with my latest mammogram results. I was meeting a friend for coffee at four.

I couldn't listen to him ramble and fumble and search for words and deliver long, convoluted sentences which take so much effort to try to follow. I couldn't listen to anecdotes I've heard countless times before.

Winter 1992–93

I tried to relax and chat over lunch, but I felt impatient. I had so much to do, including longing to be alone with my thoughts, impossible when I am with him. But just thinking this made me squirm. If I should live so long, I'll have lots of time to be alone with my thoughts.

Look at my friends Penny, Eileen, and Hannah, and my sisters-in-law, Claire and Jenny. Five widows in their fifties. Wouldn't they give anything to have Jay, Joe, Larry, Terry, and Sam back in their lives as I still have Julian? And, though I assumed my mammogram was probably fine, the ever-present possibility of recurrence surfaced and gnawed silently inside.

In Cafe Sophia my friend Connie sat across the white Formica table and looked at me, her right hand cupping her chin, her brow furrowed.

"You look tired today," she said. "What's going on?"

Two empty mugs sat on the table between us. Dried foam from decaf lattes formed a tan lacy pattern on the glass. Rock music pulsated from the coffeehouse's stereo.

"Too damn loud," I said, thinking of Julian in his nightshirt and Dr. Kushlan's pending call. Connie got up to ask Sophia to lower the volume.

Gray rain dripped outside and my legs shivered in the draft from the cafe's open door. "I feel so cold," I said. Connie left the table and quickly returned with a green wool shawl she had brought from her car. She draped it over my knees and shoulders. Still, I couldn't get warm.

"I feel sad today. . . . I'm so afraid of what's happening to Julian."

Connie looked at me and nodded.

"I keep flashing forward to when I won't be able to leave him alone. Pretty soon I'll have to make arrangements every time I want to go out."

"You've got a lot on your plate," Connie said.

"Most days I'm okay," I said. "But when I saw Julian in pajamas at noon with nowhere to go and nothing to do, I got scared."

"You know," Connie said, leaning forward on her elbows. "When I had my cancer operation, you reminded me to stay present with what's happening now. You always told me not to flash ahead to imagined problems when I got scared about a CT scan or my next X ray."

"Funny you should say that," I said. "I'm waiting for Dr. Kushlan to call about my mammogram. I'm so much better at handling cancer than Alzheimer's."

"What do you mean?"

"I mean, with my breast cancer I learned to cut off thoughts about recurrence, pain, a horrible death. I really learned not to leap ahead and imagine the worst. I'm waiting to hear about my latest mammogram. ... Sure, I'm a little nervous, but I don't obsess about it the way I do about Julian."

Connie stared at me.

"When I had my mastectomy and chemotherapy, Julian was there to help me. But his diagnosis changed that forever. ... I'm not the patient anymore. It's like I've been spared so I can care for him."

Connie nodded.

"God forbid if I should get sick. ..." I paused. "It's not everyone I can talk to when I'm afraid."

"Sometimes I think only someone else with cancer understands that fear," Connie said.

"But in some odd ways, cancer improved my life," I said. "I stopped wasting time. What's important became really clear."

"I felt that for a while," Connie said. "But it drifted away."

"Well, I still have that sense of urgency," I said. "For myself, and even more for Julian. I think my anxiety over Julian has eclipsed my fears about cancer."

Connie looked at me intently. We spoke of how isolated we feel when we're afraid, how we need friends to listen. We talked of how Julian has changed over recent weeks.

Connie told me that last Friday when we left her house after dinner, Julian walked into the back garden instead of the driveway. I told her how in the cabin at Lake Tahoe he went into friends' bedrooms returning from the bathroom in the middle of the night.

Images of Julian opening the bedroom doors of sleeping couples made us laugh. I smiled at Connie, my tall, divorced, capable friend, who lives so successfully by herself. I would be able to live alone, too, when the time came, a thought unimaginable less than a year ago. Connie was my friend . . . and she wouldn't go away, even if I told her what lay in my heart.

She stared into my eyes and I gazed into hers.

"I hear you," her eyes said.

"I hear you too," my eyes smiled back. I glanced at my watch. "Uh-oh . . . five o'clock. The doctor's office is closing. I had better call."

I removed the green shawl, handed it to her, and walked to the phone. Dr. Kushlan's nurse read me the report: mammogram normal. I sighed and returned to Connie, giving her my dad's thumbs-up sign. Connie grinned back. We zipped our parkas and left Cafe Sophia, walking out into the dark, wet parking lot to our cars. We each drove home to our separate lives and separate houses. But I felt warm now, even without Connie's shawl.

We Carry All the Shoulds in Our Shoulders

I left the house at ten after eight this morning bound for my yoga class, leaving Julian sitting at the breakfast table in his red-and-white-striped flannel pajamas. He bent over the *Chronicle* trying to comprehend the front page story about Israel accepting the return of a hundred deported Palestinians. He struggles to read any headline with the word "Israel" or "Palestinian."

"What does 'deport' mean?" he had called out as I was halfway out the door.

He asks me often these days what words mean. "What's 'judge decreed'?" he had asked earlier this morning while I was in the shower. Standing outside the glass shower door in our bathroom, he asked me four questions, each time opening the door and sticking his bearded face into the steamy stall. "Where are you going today?" he asked. And "Where's Perth?"

"I'm late for yoga, darling," I said. "I'll be right back after class. We'll have lunch together and talk then. Okay?"

I grabbed my coffee mug and fled out the kitchen door, glancing back to see him hunched over the paper, his glasses pushed up high on his forehead atop his curly gray hair.

Alzheimer's, A Love Story

I drove through fog toward the yoga class, my body tense and tight. My hip ached, my right foot hurt, and I limped as I walked from the car. I felt warm in my heavy sweatpants and sweatshirt, my body eager to lie on the pale blue mat and let tension drain away. Eager for the teacher's gentle voice and the stretches and postures which soothe me. The windshield wipers swooshed back and forth, clearing my vision.

In the class I removed my parka and tennis shoes and lay down on the mat. My back arched high off the floor, my lower back muscles tight and cramped, leaving a hollow space where my spine refused to relax. I sighed and let tension go. I breathed in deeply, held my breath, and exhaled slowly, my lower back sinking as the air escaped. Gradually my back relaxed and lay flat, loose and level with the mat.

For an hour and a half, I stretched, twisted my body into various poses, and watched my breath. Occasionally my mind flitted to tasks: call the clinic and make an eye appointment for Julian, get a ski rack for our upcoming trip to the snow, call Julian's department at Stanford to ask about his early retirement letter, remember to call the insurance company. Chores flashed in and out of consciousness, but I tried to push them away. Not push, exactly, but, rather, let them float by. Return to the breath. It's *my* time here in the yoga class, a quiet time to retreat from my brain, so filled with chatter, into my wordless body.

In "baby pose," the crinks in my ankle let go and I felt my breath begin in my abdomen and rise to my chest. In "table pose," I aligned my hands under my shoulders, knees under my hips, arching and humping my spine like a cat. In "dog pose," I lengthened my legs, shoved my hips high in the air and, with quivering arms, held my torso up off the mat. Breathing in. Breathing out. Muscles that wobbled gradually strengthened. Tight, constricted muscles relaxed and stretched.

By the session's end, for the concluding meditation, I lay peaceful on my mat, soft and loose, kinks gone. Even my sore foot didn't hurt. Could I achieve this peace if Julian were in my yoga class?

Arriving home at ten-thirty A.M., I found Julian still in his red and white pajamas. He had added his maroon velour bathrobe, and he stood at the sink washing a cup, the kitchen "sort of" cleaned. Some breakfast dishes were washed, but a cup, bowl, spoon, and two place mats remained on the table. The milk was back in the fridge, but two jam jars were out.

"Hi, darling," I said.

Julian turned and began talking, but I couldn't understand what he meant. He asked me questions, but I wasn't sure what he was asking. As I headed into the bedroom to change my clothes, he followed me, chattering on.

"You know, the library, no, not the library, the lab, you know that place, that other place where we can't go, but it's gone, all the boxes, can we go there, that other place. . . ."

I knew he was preoccupied with his lab's closing, which had finally happened last Friday. All week, scientific equipment was removed from his labs, computers and printers taken away, books boxed or thrown in recycling bins, files and papers and reprints tossed in the trash.

He had been terribly anxious. I watched him become more distraught and confused. Each time I offered to help, he shouted at me, "No! It's my business! Stay out of my business! You don't have to do my business."

One day last week Julian came home furious at something that had happened. But he couldn't explain. Later I learned from a colleague that the person responsible for cleaning the lab threw out some of his papers, concerned that he wouldn't clear his office by the deadline. Julian walked in to find his file drawers empty and his desk chair gone. The absent desk chair was the last straw.

Now, while I was changing my clothes, Julian rambled on again about the lab, the library, his keys and books. Only I couldn't understand him. I didn't get the specifics of what he was trying to say. I only understood his general confusion, his anxiety about the lab closing and having nowhere to go.

Two days after his lab and office in the medical school had closed, I had learned he must also clear out of his last remaining office. His old office in the Anatomy Building, damaged by the 1989 earthquake, had just been condemned. Julian was confused about these various rooms and grieving over his lost space. If he wasn't confused in his own mind, then he certainly was in his speech.

Taking off my sweatpants, I squeezed my eyes shut. I felt like covering my ears with my hands, but I didn't. I lay down on the bed for a minute, keeping my eyes shut tight and trying to hear him out. I didn't reason with him or explain. I didn't ask questions, I just let him talk. I tried to breathe deeply to quiet myself. All the calm I had achieved in the yoga class disappeared; my muscles were tight again and my shoulders were hunched up around my ears. Some loud critic in my head shouted: "You should be more patient!"

"Relax your shoulders," the yoga teacher had said this morning. "We carry all the 'shoulds' in our shoulders."

"Your lab *is* closed down," I finally said to Julian. "But you still have your study in the library. You can keep the faculty study even after you retire. You can always go there."

This was not the time to tell him his old Anatomy Building office must soon be vacated. Two weeks from now he must be completely out of the office where he's worked for twenty years. How were we going to accomplish that smoothly?

I lay on the bed listening to Julian ramble, taking deep breaths and releasing them slowly. I tried to let my shoulders sink from my ears and my face relax.

"It'll be okay," I told Julian. "We'll work something out. Somehow or other, it'll be okay."

But it didn't feel okay at all.

The Pain of Leaving

Two weeks after his Stanford lab was dismantled, Julian was asked to turn in the keys to his last remaining office in the old Anatomy Building. A letter arrived from the Buildings and Grounds Department:

"As of February fifteenth," it said, "the locks will be changed and no one will be allowed in the Anatomy Building."

He didn't take it well. His mouth drooped and he repeated anxiously, "Where'll I go? What'll I do?"

Julian's plan had been to move from the med school office (where he had been just a short time since the 1989 Loma Prieta earthquake) back to the damaged building where his office had been for over twenty years. He had hoped to stay there as a "professor emeritus," even after his lab closed.

The wood-paneled walls . . . his floor to ceiling bookcase filled with books, journals, and reprints collected over his thirty-year career . . . the new maroon carpet we had bought just before the quake—all remained pretty well intact.

And Julian still had keys to this building, even though it had been condemned. His labs and research offices, some ten rooms in all, existed pretty much as they did after the quake. Plaster from the ceiling lay in heaps on desktops and tables. White dust covered equipment. Floors were strewn with papers, lab coats, bottles, and tools abandoned, only the most valuable items removed. Stanford hadn't yet decided what to do with this building, so they surrounded it with yellow tape proclaiming "no admittance" and let it be.

Only Julian continued to go there. For the past two years, as he withdrew more and more from his professional life, he had sought refuge in his old office. He went there to sit quietly alone, "to think," he told me, or "to write his autobiography," or "to be away from the phones." Lately he went to "clean and sort papers."

But I knew he went because that's where he had gone for twenty years. His bike just traveled there. His body belonged in that rust-colored swivel chair, leaning back, with his feet propped on the battered gray metal desk over which hung four Chinese prints of flowers from each season, given him by a grateful graduate student from Taiwan.

Across from his desk hung a blackboard, which used to be covered with statistical formulas and research project outlines. Now it listed events from Julian's youth in Glasgow, notes for his autobiography.

Two furry rats, one mounting the other, glued on a piece of driftwood, a birthday gift from a friend, still sat above the sink. A plastic cube with photos of our three children sat in the center of his desk, which was strewn with papers, reflecting his vain attempt at choosing and discarding thousands of papers accumulated during his long career.

"Things will work out, Julian," I continually reassured him. "It's hard to retire. But we'll find new things to do. You'll see," I said repeatedly, reminding him of friends who'd retired, trying to hide the lump of fear I felt myself over what he could do.

Within a few days he seemed reconciled to the Anatomy Building's closing, though he went there daily to "sort papers."

"You select the files and books you want to keep," I said. "I'll bring boxes and we'll put them in our garage or in your study at home."

To encourage him, I bought a new floor-to-ceiling bookshelf to hold his things. But, as February fifteenth drew closer, every time I mentioned boxes, he got mad. Each time I explained that we could put his books in the car and bring them home, he shouted, "It's my business! You think I can't handle my own work? Stay out of my business!"

February 13 ... February 14 ... February 15. I knew he couldn't manage the job alone. So that Sunday I found five cartons at Safeway, and Julian and I drove to Stanford. I carried the boxes into his office. But as I placed the first book into a box, Julian shouted, "Get out of here! Leave it alone! It's my stuff! You think I'm no good! It's my business!"

I tried over and over to explain, as simply as I could, why we needed to clean the office, why we should leave it tidy as a matter of pride. But no matter what I said or how I said it, he kept saying, "Stanford will do it. Stanford will do it."

He couldn't explain himself. I very much doubted that "Stanford" would pack and move his books to his library study, or to our house, but he insisted. We stood in his dust-covered office, with papers and books piled on his desk, couch, chairs and carpet, and yelled at each other.

"Leave me alone!" he shouted. "Get out of my business!"

"You never understand what I'm saying!" I shouted back.

"They'll do it! They'll do it!"

"You don't understand anything!" I screamed in frustration.

Then, suddenly, I "got it." I didn't have to clean his office. It didn't really matter what happened to the stuff, either the books and papers he wanted to take or the ones he was leaving. It certainly wasn't imperative that Julian leave a clean office when the rest of the building was a shambles.

"Okay, okay," I said. "You're absolutely right. It's not my job to clean your office. I'm leaving. I'm not coming here again. Do whatever you want." And I just let go.

Calming down, I realized I had several options: Do nothing. Or call the secretary and see what the department might do. Or go back myself and clean up after Julian turned in the keys. I didn't have to stay and fight.

Looking back, though, I saw that I didn't let go soon enough. I could have avoided that whole scene if I hadn't tried to "reason" with Julian, to "explain," to try to get him to see it my way. How slowly I learned. So many ugly scenes before I remembered.

Julian and I walked down the long dusty corridor of the Anatomy Building for the last time. I tried to remove "Dr. Julian Davidson," the little wooden sign screwed into his door, but I couldn't find a screwdriver. I tried to peel "Dept. of Physiology" from the office door, but it wouldn't come off. I grabbed a thick *Gray's Anatomy* and two bound volumes of Julian's collected reprints of published articles and headed for the car. I didn't look back.

Outside, in the parking lot, I reached for him, my voice hoarse from shouting.

"You think I'm no good," he said. "You think I'm useless, that I can't do anything!"

"Darling"—my eyes filled with tears—"I didn't say that. I never used those words. You're saying that."

I held him against me, his body stiff and unyielding. Then his body softened and relaxed and began to shake with silent sobs.

"Cry, darling," I said. "It's okay to cry." And we stood in the parking lot holding each other and weeping.

Such a blessed release, crying together, sharing the same sorrow at the same time. A moment to cherish, not to work so hard to avoid.

"My darling man," I said. "It's sad to leave, Julian. It's sad what's happening to our life. But we're in this together. We'll do the best we can."

His body softened and he let me hug him. We drove home in silence, and once in the house we each went our separate ways for a while. He disappeared into his little study next to our bedroom to "sort papers." I puttered in the kitchen preparing supper.

And that night, in bed, we held each other close in the dark.

Removing Chains

Snow blocked the view from each cabin window, curtains of white so high, only a few inches of light shone in over the top. Pine trees were covered and deck rails obliterated. Nothing but white. A continuous shower of flakes drifted down. Suddenly the radio announced that Highways 89 and 80 were open for the first time in three days. Roads would be closed again tomorrow, as the blizzard wasn't yet over.

Seven of us—Julian and I and five friends—scurried to pack our gear and clean the cabin, trying to get out while the roads were open. For three hours Julian, the two other guys, and my friend Jan shoveled our three cars out from under huge drifts. They lifted soft, powdery snow off the cars, scraped the windows, poured hot water into frozen locks, and dug out the driveway. As soon as the snowplow cleared the road in front of the cabin, we loaded our cars and set off for home.

It had been a jolly four days, seven friends cooking together, lingering over meals, skiing cross-country through pine forests near the cabin. Lots of jokes and talk on the trail, in the kitchen, and before the fire. We had discussed animatedly the new Clinton administration, gays in the military, the prevalence of bisexuality, and whether or not lesbians choose their orientation.

As Julian and I got in the car for the long drive home, I realized we hadn't been alone together for five days, ever since we had driven to the mountains. He settled into the passenger seat while I gripped the steering wheel and eased the car along the icy road which, despite the plow, was covered with snow. I drove five miles an hour in a long line of bumper-to-bumper vehicles. Our chains clanked reassuringly as we listened to the radio weather report and ate tuna sandwiches.

"Wasn't it fun?" I asked Julian. "I had a great time, but look at this traffic," I said, watching the endless line of dark cars ahead of me as far as I could see.

On this section of road, I felt fairly confident. The road was level and the town of Truckee lay just a few miles ahead. We could get gas and coffee and inquire whether Highway 80 was open before we started over the seven-thousand-foot pass toward home. If I learned in Truckee that the road was closed, we would find a motel and stay overnight.

Driving up to the cabin, I had realized again that any trip we make, everything we do, is all up to me. Julian couldn't follow the map or the printed directions. When I got lost, he couldn't make a phone call or write down how to get there.

He was good at shoveling snow, though, and he enjoyed it, the clean, physical task of clearing the path and digging out the car while joking with friends. If only there were some physical job Julian could do with others, I thought as the car inched along in first gear.

At Truckee, I drove into the Shell station, filled the car with gas, and learned that Highway 80 was open, although chains were required over the pass. We left town, joining the long line of cars, a light snow still falling but the road clear.

Julian began talking about what he might do now that his lab was closed. Returning from trips, we often talked about the approaching weeks and what was scheduled. But this time I felt my stomach ache and my face tighten. I dreaded going home, returning to all the tasks facing me. The main job was trying to help Julian create a new life.

Julian rambled on in a disjointed way. My body tensed up, the vacation's looseness already gone.

"I haven't talked to you for four days," Julian said.

"I know, darling, I know." I confessed to myself that I had enjoyed this reprieve.

"I can't talk to the others," he said. "I can't talk fast enough."

"But you were fine, Julian. Didn't you have fun? These are our good friends."

"I couldn't talk at the table."

"Not everybody talked at meals," I said. "Didn't you see that sometimes Jerry was quiet? Wise was quiet? It's okay to be a quiet person."

How endlessly Julian and I talk about talking. So often he tells me how out-of-it he feels. I reassure him over and over that it's okay not to talk. But he can't accept it.

"You're still part of the group," I said. "Everybody loves you. Talk to one person at a time."

Tension teased across my forehead. The traffic crept along. We had already been on the road four hours. In normal traffic we would be nearly home. Here I was, trapped in a four-hour conversation with Julian with another four to go. I remembered how I used to love long car trips, when we talked without interruption. We read stories to each other and took turns driving and reading.

The traffic snaked its way up over the pass. As Highway 80 descended into the Central Valley, snow flurries eased and the road cleared. Along a straight stretch of freeway, drivers pulled cars and trucks over to a wide shoulder to remove chains.

I pulled over, too, and parked our car in gray slush. I knew Julian couldn't remove the chains, though he always used to. I had never taken off chains myself.

"Damn," I thought, getting out of the car. "I can't do it!" I looked at the long line of parked cars with men kneeling in the snow, quickly removing chains, dropping them in plastic boxes and speeding off.

Watching them, I wrestled with my thoughts. "I can't take off chains," part of me whined.

"Of course you can," whispered some new little voice.

"I can't."

"Well, try."

I knelt in the snow and examined the chains. Julian stood helplessly by the fender, his hands thrust deep in his blue parka pockets. Shushing the voice whining "Who, me? Take off chains?"

I calmly looked for some hook or fastener that would release the metal links. But I couldn't see how to unhook them. I took off my glove and groped under the fender. Furious at myself and Julian, I finally yelled, "Get in the car." I turned the car back into the line of vehicles heading down 80, listening to the chains rattling on the hard pavement.

Soon we reached another wide shoulder where cars parked. I vowed to calmly try again. If everyone else could remove their chains, why couldn't I? One or two women were even doing it. But I couldn't. I felt helpless, stupid, and angry at Julian, though I knew it wasn't his fault.

Finally a man wearing yellow rain gear walked toward us holding a sign saying "Chain Removal." Of course. And he took off the chains quickly for the small sum of ten dollars. So simple. Why had I gone through all that emotion?

Back in the car, though, Julian and I quarreled. The quarrel soon escalated into angry shouts. As I write this weeks later, I can't even remember what we argued about. I only remember shouting, feeling furious and helpless at not being able to remove the chains.

"Stupid man," ran through my brain. And pangs of guilt hit me every time I thought it.

Julian and I rehashed what had happened. Neither of us could let it go. We each needed to be right. Finally I said, "Let's just be quiet and not talk for a while." And I turned on the car radio and listened to some crackling country music full of static. Julian silently stared out the window.

"I'm sorry," I said after some minutes. "I couldn't help it. I felt so mad not being able to take off the chains. You must feel bad too."

"Why do you shout at me like that?" Julian asked softly. "I hate when you shout."

"I know, darling. I try not to. It isn't fair. I lose patience sometimes. I'm no Saint Anne, remember, only Ann."

"Can't you speak slower? Give me time to think? I can't think fast anymore. I need time for everything."

And Julian explained how slow everything feels. He said he needs more time to understand. He asked that I repeat myself.

"But can you appreciate how hard it is not to be understood?" I said.

"What's so bad about repeating yourself?" he asked.

"I'll try harder, Julian, to give you more time to follow what I say and to express yourself. I try, but I can't always do it."

I was amazed at Julian's insight, contrary to what many think about Alzheimer's patients not understanding. I explained that when I'm tired or rushed or have no time to myself, I lose patience. I told him I need time for myself each day.

"I need your help, too," I said. "I need you to help me more with chores."

"I want to help you," he said. "Tell me what to do and I'll do it."

And Julian agreed to make the bed, carry out garbage, sweep the floor, vacuum, do dishes, all those tasks he avoided for years.

"That will help a lot. I won't be so tired. I need you, Julian," I said.

"You know . . ." He paused. "One day . . . I may not be able to do anything."

I had to keep my eyes on the road, so I couldn't see his face, though his voice became husky.

"But what's the point of thinking about that?" he added quickly. "I can't do anything about it. Let's just enjoy now."

"Julian, I'll always be here, no matter what. Try to take pleasure in everything you do."

"Sometimes I think about disappearing completely," he said. "It's the most terrible thing. Who's in charge of this anyway? Wouldn't it be nice if someone knew what happens afterward? But no one in the world knows. . . . Aw . . . forget about it. Let's enjoy life."

I reached over and ruffled his hair.

"I may not be intelligent anymore, but I'm happy," he said. "I still have a good life. When I retire, there are so many things I want to do. And I'm still me."

The sky was dark now. Lights began to appear from towns sprawled along the highway, and the curving descent leveled out as the road headed straight for the Central Valley. Soon we'd be home. I felt filled with love and respect for Julian.

Neon signs—McDonald's, Burger King, Denny's—beckoned at freeway exits. Suddenly famished, we pulled off into a Burger King. Getting out of the car, I opened the rear door, lifted the metal chains from the floor where I had thrown them, and dropped them in their blue plastic box. They settled with a satisfying clank and I snapped the lid shut.

Then Julian and I walked hand in hand into Burger King, exhausted and starving, and ordered Whoppers, coffee and two large fries.

Good Times Still to Be Had

I sat on the examining table swinging my bare legs back and forth under the paper sheet. Eyeing the cold metal stirrups, I was glad to see them hanging down.

"Leave your clothing on, but take everything off below the waist," the gynecology nurse had told me, ushering me into the treatment room. "The doctor will be with you in a minute."

Nervously I glanced at the stirrups. I suddenly felt weepy and tense. At age fifty-four, having had four pregnancies, three births, and my fair share of infections, I am no stranger to the vaginal exam. They have never bothered me. Laughingly I used to joke that I would rather have a pelvic at the gynecologist's than have my teeth cleaned at the dentist's.

A knock at the door and the doctor came in, a heavyset gray-haired man, older than me. I had originally requested a woman gynecologist when I made the appointment, but she was called out unexpectedly to deliver a baby. This doctor was on call; I had never seen him before.

"What can we do for you today?" he asked, kindly enough, sitting down on the blue vinyl chair and crossing his legs, flipping through my chart, which lay on his lap.

"I need a Pap smear," I said, "and I want to talk with you about dyspareunia."

I could have said outright, painful intercourse, but this word sounded neutral. I knew it was a problem common to many post-menopausal women not taking estrogen, like me. I already guessed he would lecture me on painful intercourse being a symptom of lack of estrogen and that it could be helped by vaginal creams and lubricants. I really didn't feel like going into my whole story. I felt a knot in my stomach rising in seconds to form a lump in my throat.

"Well, let's see now," he said, putting on his rubber gloves and squeezing jelly onto the speculum. "Lie back and we'll take a look."

I lay back and placed my feet into the cold stirrups, which he had raised on each side of the table. I felt tense and gripped the table with both hands, gritting my teeth and grimacing as the speculum went in. "I never used to mind pelvic exams," I mumbled. "I never used to be so tense."

Suddenly, for no reason, I burst into tears. "Ow, ow," I yelled, my hands reaching to protect my crotch. I grabbed at his wrists. "No, no," I cried.

"We'll be done in a second," he said calmly, continuing to take the smear. Tears spilled from my eyes and ran down my cheeks. As soon as he finished, I sat up, repositioned the sheet over my knees, and rubbed the tears from my face, feeling completely foolish. He handed me a tissue and looked at me quizzically, a concerned look on his face.

"I never used to mind pelvics," I repeated. "But I get tense now, expecting it to hurt. And intercourse hurts now, most of the time."

"Vaginismus" he said. "You have vaginismus. The walls of the vagina go into spasm when you tense up and expect pain. It's a vicious circle. Tell me what else is going on," he said kindly, settling back into his chair.

And out it all tumbled. I cried and blubbered and spluttered the whole story, how my husband and I had been married thirty-two years, how we had always had a satisfying sex life, how sex had been important and gratifying in our lives. Now intercourse hurt. I avoided sex. I made excuses. I got it over with as fast as I could. It had never been like this, I said.

More tumbled out. I told him I was hardly interested in sex lately. No libido. I told him I had had breast cancer and a mastectomy four years ago, but having one breast wasn't why. I was completely comfortable with that. I told him I was taking tamoxifen for the breast cancer, an antiestrogen . . . and my husband has Alzheimer's . . . and . . . everything's changed. I broke down completely into heaving sobs.

"Well, now," he began, not overwhelmed by my torrent of words. "We have lots to talk about, don't we?"

And this fatherly white-coated stranger listened patiently as I blurted it all out. How I was losing so much: Julian as he was and my marriage as I had hoped it would be. How I grieved over our diminished life.

"For a start, you've been castrated," he said. "Tamoxifen is like castration. It deprives you of libido, sexual interest, and lubrication. The vaginal walls become dry and thin; intercourse is painful. Then fear sets in. Spasms develop and it all gets worse."

These things happened to women in *Redbook* articles and the *Reader's Digest*, I thought, not to me. Not me. I knew all this intellectually, of course, but what I realized suddenly, sitting there on his examining table, was how much it still mattered. And how much I had given up. Perhaps I didn't have to lose this part of my life so soon, even with my tamoxifen castration and Julian's Alzheimer's.

"There are things you can use." He told me about a vaginal lubricant called Replens and a new product called Astroglide. "You can also take a hot bath before intercourse and relax," he said.

I felt ridiculous, a woman married thirty-two years, priding herself on a lusty, good sex life, receiving instructions from a doctor on how to relax. "Try these suggestions and come see me in three weeks," he said.

A month later I returned to his office, and the nurse said, "Just sit down. No need to undress." When the doctor entered, I immediately apologized for my previous outburst.

"I don't know what came over me," I said, cool and controlled. "It all tumbled out."

"A lot's happening in your life just now," he said. "How has it been going?"

I told him I had taken hot baths. I told him I had tried Replens and Astroglide, to Julian's delight. "But the main thing I realized after that last appointment," I said, "was how much I still care." I had given up prematurely on a part of my life which I care deeply about and from which I can still get pleasure.

"I had just turned off," I confessed.

Yes, things have changed between Julian and me, I came to realize. I'm not turned on like I used to be. Part of it's hormonal, for sure. But an important part is in my head. I can turn myself on or off by what I think. I can acknowledge that I want lovemaking, despite Julian's Alzheimer's and all the changes in our lives. Then I must do what I need to do to make it happen. I had shut down and I didn't have to. Julian's not as eager at sixty-two as he was at forty, but he's interested enough. He's still loving and affectionate.

"There are more good times to be had," I told the doctor. "Even though it's different now."

During the past weeks I had come to understand that talking and sharing had been part of our lovemaking. Making love followed intimate conversation. Or vice versa. Now intimate talks were gone.

If Julian came to our bed at night holding the shaving cream in one hand and his toothbrush in the other, asking me if this is what he should use to brush his teeth . . . if he brought me tea in bed as he had always done, but put the tea bag in a cup of coffee or in the kettle or handed me a saucer without a cup . . . this affected how I felt. I didn't feel amorous. I felt sad. I shut off. I shut down.

For lovemaking to happen, I have to want it. I have to find those parts of Julian that still turn me on. We can put on a tape and play Baroque music. We can light a candle and caress. I can snuggle into his arms, recalling lustier times. I can remember how much I have loved him and all that he's been in my life.

I didn't tell the doctor these details. But I told him I had experimented these past weeks between the Pap smear and this follow-up visit. We spoke calmly of what I had learned.

"You've got a lot on your plate just now," he said. "And you're doing an admirable job. Call me any time that you'd like to talk."

I shook his hand and left the office. A searchlight had gone on, lighting up some dark, neglected shadows. I knew that my time with Julian was precious and that it was running out. But I understood, too, that there were good times still to be had. And whether I had them or not was largely up to me and how I thought about it.

I drove to the pharmacy and bought myself a frozen yoghurt and two more boxes of Replens.

Feeling the Alzheimer's Vise

Snuggled deep into blankets, I open my eyes, squinting at morning light which streams in through the half-drawn drapes. Beside me in bed, Julian rolls over to face me, already talking: "You know . . . we've got to get that thing . . . you know . . . the creature, no . . . the music creature from up there . . . way up there . . . the faraway one . . . the big stuff . . ."

"Hi, darling," I say. "Good morning."

"Far away . . . up there . . . the big stuff . . . the music . . ."

"You mean the concert tonight? Are you talking about the concert tonight at Memorial Church?"

"No, no . . . the faraway creature . . . big stuff . . ." He looks at me with clear blue eyes, his glasses on the bedside table.

"Are you talking about Florida? Florida is far away. You mean our trip to Florida next October?"

I roll over and lie on my back, stretch and point my toes. Taking a deep breath, I let it out slowly. "Julian, I don't know what you're talking about."

"What?" He sits up suddenly in bed. "I've said it four times! How can you not understand?"

I rack my brain for what he might mean. "Creature" is a word he often uses, a general word for any person: man, woman, or child. Not enough to go on. "Far away" he says often too. This can mean Berkeley, an hour away, where Karen lives; or Boston or New York, where Ben and Jeff live; or Florida, where we are going next fall.

It can also refer to the library at Stanford, where he sometimes still goes. "Up there" means any place that's any distance from where we are now. "Big stuff" means anyone important, in an authority position or older than Julian, as well as any important event.

I attempt more guesses, but his message, clear in his own mind, reaches no comprehension in mine. He explains again; I listen quietly.

"Oh, never mind," he says, slipping out from under the covers. "I'm going for a run." Good, I think, settling comfortably, glad for a few minutes alone before starting breakfast.

Julian strips off his pajamas and puts on his white striped office shirt and trousers, only he's forgotten underpants. He sucks in his stomach, pulls open the waistband of his pants, and points inside. Extending his index finger, he jabs in his trousers with a bewildered look on his face.

"Oh, Julian, your underpants—they're in the drawer." I point toward his dresser. He begins searching in the bookcase near the bed.

"Julian, the dresser . . . the drawer. Your underpants are in the drawer." He looks around the room in every direction except where I'm pointing. "The drawer, Julian, the drawer," I repeat, my pitch rising slightly.

"What are you mad about?" he says.

Julian responds immediately to my tone of voice and facial expression, more than to my words. He is exquisitely sensitive to my feelings. If I get angry, he gets upset. If I'm calm and patient, he is relaxed. "Mirroring," the Alzheimer's books call it.

Throwing off the blankets, I pad over to his dresser, sighing. No clean underwear is there, so I say, "Oh, I forgot, they're in the dryer."

He looks at me blankly.

"The dryer. The dryer . . . you know, next to the washing machine. . . . Go to the kitchen. . . ."

Julian goes into the bathroom and calls out, "Not here!"

He follows me down the hall, across the family room, through the kitchen to where the dryer stands. I open the door and scoop out a heap of clothes, dumping them on the dryer top.

"Here you go." I hand him clean underpants and he drops his trousers and slips them on. "Oh yeah," he says.

Back in the kitchen, as I make coffee and oatmeal, Julian says, "Guess I'll run later." He tears the blue plastic top off the Black Mountain water bottle that's just been delivered and removes the empty bottle from its stand, setting it on the floor. Then he hoists up the new full bottle and positions it on top of the white ceramic water holder.

"Julian, turn it over," I call from the sink. "Turn it upside down."

"Be quiet," he orders.

"Here, let's do it together," I say, going to him. "It's heavy." I attempt to help him take the upright bottle down from its perch, gesturing overturning it, but Julian pushes me away, saying, "I can do it, I've done it for years. I just forgot."

"You do forget sometimes. That's okay." I return to pour coffee grounds into the filter.

We both put breakfast things on the table. A brown crusty loaf of bread sits on the cutting board, and Julian begins sawing at it with a spoon.

"Get a knife, Julian," I say, quickly adding, "never mind, I'll get it."

Sitting at the table over coffee and oatmeal, we divide the morning paper. He focuses on a three-column photo of black-hatted Hasidic Jews bearing the coffin of the Orthodox Jewish teenager who was shot a few days ago. He pushes his glasses high up on his forehead and squints at the headline.

"Casket?" he asks. "What's 'casket'? How come the papers use all these weird words?"

As I explain about the funeral, the teenagers being shot, and the big demonstration in New York, he stares at me intently.

It's about time to leave for my morning walk. Taking a small piece of paper, I print at the top:

Tues. March 8. 9:30 — Bud. 10 — music class.
12 — lunch. 6 — home. 7:15 — Penny, concert.

Showing him the note, I try to describe today's schedule. I've learned to include nothing but essentials, to say no more than is necessary, using the simplest sentences I can.

But he's all mixed up between Bud and Penny, between the music appreciation class and the concert. It's now 8:55 A.M. and I'm late for my walk. Thrusting the note into his hand, I dash out the door, calling, "Remember to come home before six ... before six ... have a good day, darling. I've got to run." I vow to make tomorrow's note shorter. Leaving Julian at the breakfast table staring at the note, I wonder how much longer I'll be able to leave him alone.

Outside on the street, I take deep gulps of air and slowly exhale, my shoulders sinking with each breath. Julian can't remember that his underpants are in the dresser, yet he usually remembers to come home on time. He doesn't know the location of wall plugs when he tries to vacuum, yet he knows how to go alone to the library. He's capable in some areas, impaired in others. His abilities fluctuate from day to day, maddeningly inconsistent. It's exhausting being vigilant and trying to assess each situation. It's all so puzzling.

Striding past the eucalyptus, I think how our talks have become a mockery of conversation. Julian and I sometimes "converse," only no information is exchanged. He speaks. I listen and respond, "Uh-huh, that's interesting, no kidding." He speaks again. "I didn't know that," I might say. We perform the "dance" of conversation: talking, listening, responding; talking, listening, responding. And he seems satisfied with our exchange.

I understand best when I already know what he's trying to say; it's nearly impossible to comprehend new information. Sometimes I tell him simply, "Julian, I don't understand what you mean." If I say it gently, he sometimes tries again or shrugs his shoulders, saying, "Oh, never mind. I'm tired." Or, "It's late." Or, "I'll tell you later." His repertoire of phrases helps him save face.

But he often needs to tell me something. Someone called, maybe, or something happened. And I must struggle to guess and strain for the elusive meaning of his vague cues. Sometimes I need to tell him to be home at a certain time or what's happening tonight. Nothing is easy anymore. No communication can I take for granted.

Yet occasionally we have surprisingly meaningful talks.

Yesterday, driving to the market, we spoke of friends in Oregon who may get divorced. The man has moved out, separating from his wife of thirty years. I told Julian he's having a midlife crisis and wants a trial separation.

"Is there another woman?" Julian's remark startled me. "How sad," he said. "After all those years. They seemed happy."

Tears sprang to my eyes as I thought of these friends I've known since college; we've kept in touch and traveled together. Now her husband no longer loves her and claims she hasn't loved him. She is devastated and feels betrayed and unloved.

My voice caught in my throat as I stammered, "I feel so bad for Marge."

Julian reached over and laid his hand on my knee, and I brushed away tears that blurred my vision.

"No matter what happens, Julian," I said, "we've loved each other."

"Poor Marge," he went on. "I know we'll always be together." My heart split open: this startling fragment of talking intimately as man and wife. Each of us knew we were deeply loved. I marveled at how connected Julian was on an emotional level. Despite his severe language problems, Julian still revealed amazing flashes of insight.

Returning home to our courtyard, through the kitchen window I see Julian at the sink washing dishes. As I enter, he says, "Where's the stuff . . . the big stuff . . . not your big stuff . . . my other stuff . . . the one that's different?"

I push my arms against the kitchen wall, bend one knee, and extend my left leg, stretching my calf muscles. I'm silent, mulling over what he might mean.

"Well, say something," he snaps. "The other big stuff . . . where the creature . . ."

"Julian, I'm not following you."

"You think I'm no good." He throws down the sponge and leaves the room.

In the solitude of my shower, I feel it all: utter frustration at not understanding him; despair over Julian not understanding my simplest remarks; grief at losing my clever, empathetic, interesting husband; sadness over the isolation I increasingly feel. How can I stay patient as this Alzheimer's vise presses in from all sides?

"I can't keep this up," I mutter to myself as hot water sprays my back. "How do caregivers get enough strength?"

Back in our bedroom, as I'm getting dressed, Julian puts on his jacket and waits for his friend Bud to pick him up. They're going to a music appreciation class at the Jewish Community Center and then out to lunch. Julian is whistling "If I Were a Rich Man" from *Fiddler on the Roof*. His face looks relaxed, he seems for now to have forgotten about "the big stuff" and "the creature far away."

I go to him, press my face against his bristly beard, and hug him tight. Our hug lingers a few seconds longer than usual, and I feel his heavy weight against me.

Spring 1993

I want to love the flower,
even past its fullest bloom.

I Want to Speak of Fog and Flowers

I fold the pillow in half this time and sit cross-legged, settling my hips on the pillow's edge. I wad up my sweatshirt, placing it under my right thigh. Maybe my leg won't hurt so much this way. It's the last "sit" of the Zen Buddhist weekend Julian and I are attending.

Ding. Ding. Ding. The bell rings three times, announcing the start of this meditation. Its clear tone shimmers out like ripples on the surface of a pond. In two short days I've come to love this sound. Time to wake up. Another chance to be aware.

The rustling of clothes from people adjusting their posture has stopped. Around the room, twenty people sit cross-legged on the floor, facing the wall. Julian sits next to me on my right, a lanky dark-haired woman in white pants and an olive green shirt sits to my left.

The Zen Buddhist priest with his shaved head and black robes sits in the lotus position at the front of the room. Although I can't see him during the meditations, I feel his presence.

My right leg is comfortable so far. I say "so far" because my right leg has pained me in previous sits. I'm prepared for it to hurt and I'm not surprised when it does. But I am surprised when it doesn't. I notice that nothing hurts just now. I feel comfortable — and I know it won't last.

Sure enough, now I have a hot burning sensation in my right knee. Now it moves along my shin bone. Now down the back of my thigh. I try to sit still and just let it be, to breathe into the pain, maybe ease it. It doesn't help. I lower my right knee, let it sink, give it over to gravity. I feel some tendon stretch and release.

Now I'm aware that my shoulders are hunched up toward my ears. I let them relax. Thirty minutes is a long time to sit. If I'm tense or tight, I can't do it. I must find the most comfortable position and make minute adjustments as new discomforts come and go.

Through half-open eyes I see the chalk white wall before me, with irregular swirls of plaster. A tan baseboard runs a few inches above the carpet, blue-gray with a short nap. I see my knees and shins in my black pants. The only sounds: a bird's chirp, an occasional cough, someone clearing his throat, and the rustling of Julian's nylon gym pants as he changes position.

Julian gets up on his knees and leans on the wall. No one else moves. He settles himself. I'm aware of him moving and I try to refocus attention on my breathing.

I follow my breath: Inhale, exhale. Inhale, exhale. Slower, slower. Deeper, deeper. Follow the breath. Inhale: my belly softens and swells, then my chest expands as air fills it, then chest and belly relax. When I follow my breath, I don't feel so much pain in my leg, nor do I care so much what Julian is doing.

My eyelids drop and close. It's easier to focus when my eyes are closed, but Reb Anderson, the Zen priest leading the retreat, has told us to keep them open. It will be easier to carry this feeling into daily life, he says, if we meditate with eyes open. After just two days I look forward to these meditations, hard as they are, instead of dreading them.

Thoughts float by—where's Julian, has he gone to the bathroom, what position is he in, do his noises bother the others, should I have explained to Reb Anderson why Julian is the only person who doesn't sit in the traditional position and who doesn't hold his hands in the suggested "mudra"? Thoughts come and go. I try to let them float by, to notice them and let them pass. I open my eyes, stare at the white wall, and return to following my breath.

Ding. Ding. Ding. The clear tones ring out, sweet and pure. Slowly I uncross my stiff legs, flex and extend my feet, and stand up, letting the ache ease out of my joints. I turn around to see other people adjusting themselves on their pillows. We all face center, where lavender, purple, and white stock bend out of a tall glass vase.

Reb Anderson sits back on his legs and smiles. His shaved head and black robes have dominated my attention these past two days. I've stared and stared at him. But it's not just his shiny scalp and robes that fascinate me, it's his face. His clear blue eyes watch intently as each person speaks. His smile, his laugh, his frown, his silence and stillness seem as clear as the meditation bell.

As he answers questions I am riveted to his face and words. Yet my thoughts wander too.

Alzheimer's, A Love Story

How odd that I am here. It was Julian who found this retreat advertised on a flyer. He wanted to come and I did not. But how deeply meaningful this experience has become. I feel like a dried sponge soaking up water. The meditations, the slow walking, the "dharma talks," our questions and Reb's answers—I can't get enough. Strangely, I am not offended nor do I feel resistant to what he says, as I so often do in Jewish services—or Christian—or so many of the "religious" situations I've experienced.

I don't understand what he says much of the time. It's puzzling and complicated and often seems convoluted. He uses long sentences which I can't follow. But I am intrigued. I am open to him. I am full of awe and wonder. I am moved by Reb's compassion and his presence.

I think of myself and Julian. I think of acceptance. If I can be mindful in each moment, I believe I will experience less anxiety and grief. When I opened the dishwasher three days ago and saw two loaves of bread on the rack, I was startled. If I had just observed, "Oh, Julian's put the bread in the dishwasher," then I would simply experience that moment that way, instead of being upset.

"Stay present," the Buddhist priest says. "Moment by moment."

How helpful this could be to Julian too. Morning after morning, night after night, he obsesses over what he "should do." Over coffee on our oak breakfast table, or snuggled under the blankets at night, he says, "I've got to find something to do. I need to think about what I can do."

"Listen to this beautiful music," I tell him, putting a Brandenburg concerto into the tape deck. Or, "Look how blue that ceanothus is," or, "Take a walk, darling, and enjoy the lupine and poppies on Cowhill."

If only he could slow down and stop his mind from struggling over what he could "do." If only he could simply "be." He can walk down a path through a redwood forest, sit on a sand dune gazing out at the sea, swim in the pool, ride his bike, and listen to music with as much enjoyment as any man.

"Be mindful of the present moment," Reb Anderson says. And I vow to try.

In this closing session Reb reads a poem. Across the room in my direct line of vision is a large plate glass window. Outside hangs thick fog. I can't see the sloping green hill, the redwood grove, or the checkered fields I saw yesterday when the sky was clear. Today I see only a light gray curtain of fog.

As Reb reads the poem I stare through the window at the fog. Suddenly a dark redwood emerges out of the mist. Then another. Fog blows away, revealing five dark trees, as if someone has drawn back a curtain. I'm startled to see them. Then, as quickly as they appeared, they are gone.

Reb asks each person in the workshop to say a few words. It's my turn to speak. I haven't planned anything.

"I want to speak of fog," I begin slowly. "And flowers." Twenty pairs of eyes turn my way.

"I've never been to a meditation retreat before," I say. "I haven't understood much of what you've said, Reb. Some of your words have been like a mysterious fog. From time to time I've glimpsed some shape I recognize, then I lose it." And I describe the redwoods that just emerged, then disappeared in the fog.

"And the flowers," I say, focusing on the white and lavender stock bending out of the vase in the circle's center, "are a powerful image."

I told the group in the opening session that Julian and I had both been diagnosed in recent years with life-threatening illnesses. I said we were looking for ways to calm ourselves and experience more love and peace.

Reb spoke to us the second day of flowers.

"A flower is perfect, just as it is," he said. "First the tiny green shoot pushes up from the earth. Then a stem grows and leaves unfold. Then a bud forms, gradually opening into the flower. The flower blooms for a time, its petals wide open, its color intense, its stem sturdy. Each flower has its time of enhanced blooming. Then, slowly, the stem droops a little, the flower's color darkens, petals begin to drop. This is the way of flowers."

I stare at the purple stock and my voice quivers. Julian sits in a half-lotus position on the rug beside me and I worry fleetingly what he feels about what I'm saying.

"I want to love the flower," I continue, "even past its fullest bloom."

Reb sits solidly on his round black cushion, each foot resting on the opposite thigh, his hands motionless on his knees. His clear blue eyes focus intently on me, and he smiles.

Learning to Live With Alzheimer's

"Where's my or . . . ortha . . . o-dee . . .?" The day begins. I'm lying in bed snug under my flowered spread, dozing, relaxing, letting the new day wake up.

"Where's my o-dee?" Julian repeats, standing at the foot of the bed wearing a shirt and underpants, holding one shoe in his hand. He searches for the word. "I can't find that thing, that blue thing that, you know, he's helping me with, that flat thing to read with." He means "walk with."

"Orthotic," I say. Julian's podiatrist has given him special soles for the arthritis in his feet. We've already lost and found them several times over the weekend. I slide out from the warm bed and locate them in his black tennis shoes, which I had remembered seeing in the family room under the couch.

In the kitchen I start laying out breakfast. Julian suddenly appears wearing a huge pair of pants.

"Hey! What's going on here?" He holds up the gaping waist. "What is this? My pants don't fit!"

I'm shocked. He's wearing my father's pale blue trousers which I've just washed and hung on a hanger on a doorknob. He's put them on, not even realizing they weren't his.

A few months ago I would have been horrified. I would have cried. I would have been haunted by that image of Julian wearing my father's pants three sizes larger than his and a color he's never owned. I would have anxiously described the incident to friends.

"They're my father's pants," I laugh. "I do Dad's laundry." It's over in a minute. I'm getting used to Julian's odd behavior; mercifully we can learn to adjust.

Dressed in his own pants and shoes with the orthotics inside, Julian returns to the kitchen for breakfast. He used to make coffee, but he's had a hard time ever since our Mr. Coffee broke last month and we've returned to pouring boiling water into a funnel set over the thermos. He has to heat water in the kettle first. All the objects are different: red thermos and black filter instead of a glass pot and white filter.

"Where's that thing?" It's hard for Julian to locate the necessary equipment. Finding objects requires visualizing what's needed before he can search. Maybe this explains why he often has a puzzled look on his face, examines countertops, or meanders from room to room. He's looking for something, only he doesn't remember what, just as Nancy Mace, author of *The Thirty-Six-Hour Day*, described.

I glance up from setting the table to see him pouring boiling water into the funnel. Only he's forgotten to put it over the thermos. Brown liquid seeps out from under the funnel onto the counter.

"Whoa!" I say. "Here's the thermos." I swoop up the funnel and place it over the thermos, wiping the spreading coffee with a sponge. Today, for some reason, it's no big deal. I feel relaxed. It's even funny and I laugh.

Why today am I not upset when on other days, events like these make me snap, mutter, and feel tense, angry, and scared? I realize I'm learning to handle things differently. Reviewing many upsetting situations, I've become aware of my thoughts in the midst of hard times. I've learned to track that flash of reaction between situation and upset, to discover my intervening thoughts.

When Julian does something odd, I sometimes think, "Stupid man!", "Oh God, he's getting worse!" or "I'm going crazy." These thoughts flash through my brain, faster than I'm aware of them. But when I stop and tell myself, "The man I love has terrible memory problems," or, "He can't help it," I react differently and better feelings emerge. Replacing harsh statements with more helpful ones changes the way I feel.

Events alone don't create bad feelings. What we think and tell ourselves causes a large part of our distress. I can't control what Julian says and does; I *can* control how I react.

Finally Julian is ready to leave. He hops on his bike and pedals off to the library, leaving me facing the breakfast clutter. I sigh and my shoulders sink two inches as the swirl of energy surrounding Julian's departure settles down. I feel like Blondie shoving Dagwood Bumstead out the door.

I lean back in my chair to finish my coffee and think back to yesterday's session in the New Couples' Group. "Nothing dramatic happened," I had said when it was my turn to report. "But each day is filled with irritating events."

I commiserated with Bill, whose wife has Alzheimer's. He had just described how he broke down and cried after an incident at the dentist's office. Fatigue and loss overwhelmed him, and he despaired at the endless frustrating situations.

Tears filled my eyes as he described going into his car and crying. Bill felt real to me yesterday, as never before; previously he had seemed distant, stoic, and controlled. I felt close to him, this man with whom I would probably have little in common outside the group.

"Yes, yes," I had said. "It's all these incidents, day after day."

As I spoke Julian stared at me with pain in his eyes. He looked hurt and anguished.

"Maybe I shouldn't have said that." I apologized quickly.

"I didn't know you were suffering," Julian said. "Stop worrying. I don't worry. I just want to live my life." He looked hard at me. "You don't need to worry about the future."

"Yes," I blurted out, "but I'm doing everything so you *can* live your life. *I* worry, plan, and make endless arrangements. You don't even realize what I do."

As soon as the words left my mouth, I regretted them. Do I need Julian to thank me? To be grateful? To be aware of all I do? Yes, sometimes. Selfish and immature, perhaps, to expect recognition, but that day I needed it. I wanted acknowledgment.

A current of connection ran around the group. I saw it in everyone's eyes. Looking from face to face, I saw our common struggle. I felt close to each memory-impaired person struggling to go on living a meaningful life despite ever-increasing limitations. And close to each Alzheimer's spouse, the second victim. We each do the best we can; we keep on going. We hold our "normal life" in a sieve while it drips slowly away.

Sipping my coffee and staring at the cluttered kitchen

table—I realize that it's in these awkward acts of daily living that I experience Alzheimer's. I remember the first months after Julian's diagnosis—I was depressed, terrified, angry, and sad. What I've learned over the past two years has helped, even as Julian's competence steadily shrinks.

It's interesting that Julian never talked about ending his life. Early on, I had worried he might. A writer he admired, Arthur Koestler, committed suicide, after learning he had leukemia and Parkinson's, together with his wife. It seems most Alzheimer's patients do not take their own life. Perhaps it is because when they can plan and carry out this act, they are in good enough shape not to want to. And when they may want to, they no longer can. It is a complex subject. But Julian refused to dwell on what might happen later and mostly focused on pleasures and activities he could still do, for which I am grateful.

I finish my coffee and carry dirty dishes to the sink.

A line from a Beatles' song pops into my head: "It's getting better. . . ."

I hum the tune quietly as I place dirty cups in the dishwasher. My life doesn't hurt as much as before. Maybe because I've given up yearning for the life I had expected. I understand that it's not to be. After resisting and flailing against the changes, I grow closer to accepting.

Julian is definitely getting worse. But in some odd way, I am getting better. Not every day, for sure, but at least I feel better this morning.

The Courage to Adjust

Tomorrow Julian and I go to the Duveneck Ranch to work in their garden.

"Drive down the dirt road along the stream," the volunteer coordinator said on the phone. "The garden's on your right. Look for a tall, gray-haired man with a ponytail, named Andy."

I had called the ranch last week after hiking there with a friend. The Duveneck family had for generations owned hundreds of acres of oak-studded hills. They developed hiking trails for public use and opened up their farm so that children could visit. Their mission is to introduce city kids to nature and share their land with the community.

Ambling down the moist path that followed a cascading stream, I felt so peaceful. Purple lupine lined the trail and wild blue iris poked up through lush beds of miner's lettuce. Ferns washed clean by the drought-ending rains brushed our jeans, and thick redwoods stood by the trail, the rust-colored bark cool and damp under my hand's touch.

If only Julian could spend time in this beautiful place, I thought. As I headed back to my car parked near the garden, I saw teenagers sitting in dark brown earth between lettuce rows, weeding. Maybe there's work here that Julian could do.

I remembered our trip to the Northwest last fall, when we'd visited Mark on Bowen Island and a friend who lives in the woods outside Bellingham, collecting bark and berries for her potpourri business. I remembered the lawyer with Alzheimer's we had met in the couples' group, who volunteers in the Santa Cruz arboretum.

If only Julian could do physical work outside, I thought, in a beautiful place. Living on a university campus among high-powered intellects, and sitting for hours in the Stanford library, when he can neither read nor write, is somehow going in the wrong direction. I know he's comforted to maintain his familiar routine of visiting the library, editing papers, and carrying his bulging green briefcase back and forth. But how calm he might feel if he did activities that didn't require words.

Julian had worked on a farm in England for three years as a teenager, preparing to go to Israel and live on a kibbutz. He's told me stories of cutting hay with a scythe and milking cows. Not only does Duveneck Ranch have a garden, they have horses, goats, sheep, and a cow. I called the ranch office when I got home from the hike.

The volunteer coordinator listed various jobs volunteers can do: gift shop, nature center, leading school children around the farm. When I explained that my husband is a retired Stanford pro-fessor with Alzheimer's, she immediately said, "Oh, come on

Wednesdays and work in the garden. Planting, weeding, picking. There are different jobs all year round."

"My husband will need supervision," I said. "He can't really work alone. He forgets what to do."

"Andy's always there," she said. "He's very patient. Developmentally disabled adults from a special school also volunteer. Andy's used to working with special folks." Her voice was kind and welcoming. "It must be hard for you," she added.

My eyes filled with tears hearing her speak. I envisioned Julian working in the garden. Maybe I could work there too. Of course I would take him the first few times.

"Bring food," the volunteer coordinator said, "to share for lunch. After work, everyone eats together."

Then she said, "You may be interested to know that we're thinking of organizing some respite weekends on the ranch for Alzheimer's patients to give their families a break. Maybe two or three times a year. It's just in the planning stage."

I couldn't believe my ears. Incredible how one thing leads to another, how seemingly haphazard events come together. I had hiked at the Duveneck Ranch with a friend, thought about Julian's needs, and now this new work was before us.

Julian was excited when I told him. "Did you phone the farm?" he kept asking. And when I told him we were going on Wednesday, he said, "I'm so excited." He has asked every day since, "When do we go?"

"Tomorrow," I told him. "We go to the ranch tomorrow."

I hope it works. I hope Andy is nice and that Julian likes it. Maybe we'll learn to make compost. Maybe we'll make a garden at home.

I think of our new, quiet life: yoga, music appreciation, walking, meditating. How small and immediate our life has become.

Yesterday I wrote a colleague of Julian's who invited him to the annual conference of the International Academy of Sex Research, one of his former professional organizations. He's going to receive an award. I wrote to explain Julian's state: that he's forgotten all he knew about science, that no one should talk to him about anything professional, that he can hardly read or write. I wanted to prepare her for how he's changed in the three years since she's seen him. But writing her reminded me of his previously high-powered life and made me sad.

Would she think, "How pathetic that Julian is now excited over weeding a garden?" Or would she understand the courage and resilience required to adjust, accept, and search out the next new thing? It doesn't matter what she thinks. It's me who flip-flops from thinking how small and puny our life is to how mellow and satisfying these quiet acts can actually be.

Tomorrow we go to the garden.

The Kindness of Strangers

As I drove down the freeway toward the Duveneck Ranch, Julian said, "I'm so excited. Remember the farm . . . I cut with . . . a . . . that thing."

"A scythe. Yes, I know that story. When you were sixteen, you cut alfalfa on the kibbutz. But remember, this isn't a kibbutz or a big farm. We'll be working in a small vegetable garden."

We turned off the freeway just ten minutes from our house and headed west into hills heavy with oak trees, manzanita, flowering madrone, and bright yellow Scotch broom. The road twisted and curved past corrals holding chestnut and sorrel horses, past apple trees whose dark branches sparkled with white blossoms.

"We're just twelve minutes from our house," Julian said looking at his watch.

Finally I saw the small wooden sign: "Duveneck Ranch — Hidden Villa. Farm and Wilderness Preserve." I turned in, following the dirt road to the parking lot. We got out of the car and walked toward the garden, past a hillside luxuriant with ferns, miner's lettuce and tender new poison oak, bright green after the rains.

The garden stretched to our right, roughly an acre, row after row planted with vegetables surrounded by yellow marigolds and white and purple cosmos. Three scarecrows stood by the fence, and silver metal strips dangling from a wire flapped in the breeze.

"Look at those shiny things," Julian exclaimed, his eyes lighting up as the silver strips danced and glistened in the sun.

Spring 1993

In the garden two men wearing jeans and denim workshirts pushed wheelbarrows to the newly plowed beds. An older man with white hair, a young man in his twenties, and two women about my age spread rich dark compost onto the earth with pitch-forks. I had a fleeting moment of doubt.

Would Julian like this? Would he get bored or do the wrong thing? What did I know about farming anyway? But before I had time to sink into hesitation, a lanky teenager wearing denim over-alls with a baseball cap set backward over his black dreadlocks walked toward us.

"Hi," he waved. "I'm Aiza."

"Hi," I answered, uncertain of what he had said. "Aida?"

"Aiza." he repeated. "With a 'z.'"

"I know two Aidas and one Aisha," I said, "but no Aizas. We're Julian and Ann, come to help in the garden. Is Andy here?" I looked about the garden for the gray-haired man with a ponytail.

"Andy's taking a sick goat to the vet. He'll be back soon. I'm his assistant. You here to volunteer?"

"Did Andy tell you we would be coming?" The volunteer coordinator had told me she would alert Andy about Julian's Alzheimer's so he could explain slowly and clearly what we were to do. I hoped Aiza knew, too, so it would be less awkward.

"No," he said. "But come on. I'll show you what we're doing. Take this." He pointed to a wheelbarrow and handed Julian and me two digging forks. "Go to the next field, fill this with compost, and then spread the compost on these beds." Aiza stood in a nar-row furrow between two wide raised mounds of earth.

Julian lifted the handles of the wheelbarrow and pushed it straight across the carefully worked earth. The front wheel left a deep track, and Julian's tennis shoes pressed down the raked soil, leaving dark footprints.

Oh, no, I said to myself. But Aiza handled it. "Walk here," he said softly, pointing to the furrow. "We're going to plant let-tuce in these beds." He seemed used to explaining things to novices.

Around the garden schoolchildren clustered near the compost pile, ran up and down rows of young bean, corn, and tomato plants, and admired the scarecrows. Volunteers enthusiastically pointed out earthworms and sow bugs crawling in the compost.

Julian finally maneuvered the wheelbarrow out of the bed and into the furrow, pushing it down the path toward the compost heap. I carried two digging forks, feeling self-conscious. Joining the two women and the young blond man at the compost, we stuck our forks into the rich fertilizer and lifted it awkwardly into the wheelbarrow.

The other workers greeted us warmly. "Hi," each said. "I'm Jane." "Jeannie." "Don." We all shook hands. "Wednesday's my favorite day," Jeannie said, wiping her hands on her jeans. I wondered if it would become Julian's favorite day too.

Everyone maneuvered the wheelbarrows back to the garden. Julian pushed ours, looking proud of himself. Back at the beds he spread forkful after forkful of fertilizer onto the same spot, making a thick pile in one place.

"We just need a thin layer. About an inch," Aiza said. Julian fumbled at trying to pull the wheelbarrow down the furrow to allow us to pitch compost on a new spot.

"Like this, Julian," I said, trying to keep irritation and embarrassment out of my voice. "Spread it like this." I sank my fork into the rich mixture, lifted it over the wheelbarrow's side, and gently shook it back and forth, as I copied Jane's, Jeannie's, and Don's movements.

After several trips to and from the compost, Julian announced he had to go to the bathroom. Jane pointed to a small shed across the field beyond the fence. Julian headed in the opposite direction, toward the main farmhouse, which was in his line of vision, exactly opposite from where she pointed, just as he had done when we went to the movies. His confusion about the location of places was slowly increasing. I knew he would never be able to get to the bathroom and return.

"I have to go too. We'll be right back," I said quickly, setting off with Julian to the bathroom. When we returned, the young blond man said, "Hey, Julian, come over here with me," and they unloaded his wheelbarrow together. I sighed with relief. How comforting these tiny acts of kindness.

Spring 1993

When the women and I were alone in the furrow, I said simply, "Julian has Alzheimer's. He needs repetitions to understand what he's supposed to do."

"How good that you're here," one immediately said. "I hope he likes it," said the other. The next time I was alone with Aiza, I told him too. Don had apparently guessed on his own. I felt relieved of the anxiety of their thinking Julian stupid or weird.

For two hours we unloaded compost from the wheelbarrows, walking back and forth between the fields. I figured out how to lift the digging fork without straining my back. The sun shone through a cloudy sky; two hawks circled overhead while kindergarten children and their teachers walked in groups past the garden. Marigolds and daisies made a colorful border along the edge of the furrows. Sometimes we chatted casually, sometimes we worked quietly. Julian whistled a tune from *My Fair Lady*.

Soon a tall man with a ponytail approached, holding out his hand in greeting. "Hi, I'm Andy," he said. "Everything okay? We're glad you could come."

Andy told everyone about the sick goat and then announced we would spend the last hour weeding potatoes. We all trooped into the next field, where young green plants surrounded by straw mulch grew in two straight rows on raised beds. We settled down to pulling weeds. Again Julian stepped right on the plants.

"We try not to walk here," Andy said to Julian. "These are potatoes and these are weeds," he said as Julian pulled up a small potato plant. Andy spoke kindly, simply, with patient respect. I kept my face down, focused on my weeding. But I began to realize Julian probably would not be able to work here alone without me, my original plan.

By one o'clock we had finished the potato rows. Andy had taken a small red tiller and turned the compost we had spread into the soil. "Lunchtime," he called out. Julian and I followed the others to a wooden table set in the shade of a large pine. We washed our muddy hands under a tap. Soon the table was covered with food that emerged from backpacks and the kitchen of a nearby house: potato salad, pita, veggies, hummus, fruit, cheese, French bread, and juice.

Julian and I sat somewhat self-consciously at one end of the picnic table, listening to the banter. They spoke of the sick goat, the crops to be planted, Aiza's summer plans. They asked us a few questions: how we had heard of Hidden Villa, whether we had worked in a garden before. Julian told briefly and hesitantly of working on a farm in England when he was sixteen. I felt increasingly relaxed.

"What good food," Julian said, seeming quite at ease after his remarks were accepted by the group.

At the meal's end everyone said, "Bye, Julian. Bye, Ann. Hope we see you next week." Julian and I left and I led him up the road, past a pen of white goats and a newborn kid, ironically named "Little Ann."

"Julian, I want to show you something," I said heading toward the trail I had hiked with my friend a few weeks before.

The creek trail meandered along a stream cascading over rocks, settling into quiet pools, swirling around fallen logs. Purple lupine grew in clumps along the water's edge, and ferns, young redwoods, and live oak covered the hillside.

Julian and I walked hand in hand silently along the soft path. No words were needed. His face looked smooth and relaxed. He paused from time to time and we gazed quietly at a deep pool. He looked at me and smiled. He squeezed my hand and whistled a Yiddish tune. I made a mental note to cancel the dentist appointment I had made months ago for next Wednesday. I already knew even without asking Julian that we would both come to Hidden Villa again.

What Julian Must Accept

Julian and I walked into the V.A. conference room yesterday, where Helen, the psychiatric nurse, greeted us, trim and petite in a black skirt and silk blouse brightened with a gold braided necklace.

We sat down around a wooden table. Filled with questions to ask and things to tell her, I kept quiet, wanting Julian to speak. I talk easily. I have lots to say and friends to speak to. Julian has only me.

Spring 1993

"So, what's been going on?" Helen looked straight into Julian's eyes. She waited. I waited. No one spoke. Helen just watched Julian, smiling.

"I've been thinking," Julian slowly began. "I'm not the same anymore. For a long time I thought I was, but I'm not."

I sealed my lips and watched Helen watch Julian.

"At first it was just words," he said. "I can't speak well. I thought it was only words. But it's more than that."

"You're aware of changes?" Helen asked gently.

"Yes." Julian crossed his legs and leaned forward in his chair, closer to this woman who sat ready to hear him. "I can't do what I want to do."

Haltingly, Julian told about not working since his lab and office closed. And really he wasn't active months before that. He spoke of how he had looked forward to being free: to write his autobiography, work with Amnesty International or an Israeli peace organization, travel to foreign places.

"But I can't do these things," he said.

Helen nodded and answered slowly, "It's hard to stop your work, Julian. You have the same problems most people have when they retire, only you also have serious limitations." She told him it might take a while to find things he enjoys, reminding him it's just been three months since his lab closed.

"It's a difficult transition," she said. "What kind of things are you doing?" And Helen turned to me.

I told her Julian volunteers at the Food Closet, packing eggs, flour, and peanut butter into small containers to be handed out to people in need. He sings in a Yiddish Chorus. He comes with me to yoga, meditates, and works in Hidden Villa's garden. I spoke enthusiastically about these activities we had found.

Julian's mouth turned down into a sad, thin line.

"Yes, but I need something exciting," he said. "I need exciting work. Something creative."

"It's hard to give up operating on the high level you've been used to. You must learn what you can do realistically," Helen said, adding, "It seems Ann is excited about these things, but you're not." She smiled.

Defending myself, I explained that I had tried to find things he might enjoy, saying he had long been interested in meditation and living a simple life.

"What about Siddhartha?" I asked Julian. "You admired the man who spent his last years ferrying people across the river."

"Julian's come a long way." Helen raised her arm high over her head. "He was up here," she said. Then she lowered her arm to shoulder level. "Now he's here."

Julian watched her intently with wide, soft eyes.

"He's used to a more complex life," she said. "It's hard to adjust to change."

"But it's good for him to work in the garden," I protested. "To be in nature . . . outdoors . . . doing simple tasks."

"I did that already when I was nineteen," Julian mumbled. "In that place and then in that other place, that big place."

"He means that he worked on a farm in England and Israel," I explained.

"If *you* love working in the garden," Helen said to me, "you should continue."

"Yes, but I went for Julian. I don't need more things to do. I thought he would like it."

"Julian needs time to figure out what he wants," she said, acknowledging Julian's less-than-eager response to my recounting of the life I had set up.

Julian smiled, pleased to be understood. "But," said Helen to Julian, "you need something to do *even if* it's not quite right. If you just stay home, you'll get depressed. You need to go out every day, have a schedule and do things with people. *And* keep looking for what feels right."

"Do both," she emphasized. "Keep on with what you're already doing *and* look for new activities that feel more interesting—remembering, of course, what's realistic."

I felt relieved. Julian smiled and said, "Okay, I'll go to the farm. But it's not exciting."

A lump rose in my throat. No, it's not exciting. Going to my yoga class and weeding potatoes does not equate with taking testosterone samples from a tribe living in Papua New Guinea or camping on the Masai-Mara game preserve observing hyenas or being the head of a busy research team. All that he's done, all that he's lost.

Then Julian told haltingly of the award he would receive in June at the annual meeting of the International Academy of Sex Researchers and how he wanted to say something.

"Just say 'Thank you,'" I said, telling Helen I've been saying this for weeks. "Julian thinks he has to say something professional. He's been trying to read physiology journals and it's hard for him."

I didn't say flat out, "He can't read at all," but I gave Helen a look that said so.

"You've finished your work," Helen said. "You're being honored for work already done. Just go and enjoy the award. Read journals if you want, for your own pleasure. But don't feel you need to comment or contribute scientifically."

"It's so hard to let go," I said.

"He's already let go of a lot," Helen added.

It was Helen's presence that comforted, more than her actual comments, the way she sat and listened to Julian, her willingness to witness and be present with our pain.

Julian leaned back in his chair and smiled.

"Helen," I said. "We really appreciate these talks. Most professionals don't engage with you, they don't know how to help."

"Thank you," she said slowly. Then she looked at Julian. "You have a lot to say. I learn as much from you when we meet as you do from me."

Helen turned to me. "Julian has much to teach me."

My mind jumped to last night, when Julian held me in his arms and said, "I'm not normal anymore. I used to think I was, but I'm not now. I may become a weird person who can't speak. A person nobody wants."

"I'll always be with you," I told him. "I'll always love you."

"Maybe I'll live in a hole," he said, rather casually.

"I don't know of any holes or caves around here," I said. "But you could live in the garage. We could bring in rocks and make it look like a cave and you could sit there and meditate and I'll bring you food."

And he laughed. "How lucky I am to have you," he said.

"Few families with Alzheimer's have talked or written about it," Helen said. "And, Julian, few explain their feelings as clearly as you express yours."

"Everyone must deal with hard things in life," she added. "These are the cards you've been dealt. We each have to do as well as we can."

Yes, yes, I thought. Clichés, maybe, but her words sank deep. I felt understood and inspired to give it my best.

I saw Helen's face, soft and filled with compassion. I realized help was out there, though the burden was surely mine. I hoped I would be strong enough to do what needed to be done . . . and my love for Julian deep enough to see me through what lay ahead.

"You're doing a very important job," I said to Helen.

"So are both of you," she answered.

Her simple words somehow made me feel acknowledged and not so alone. The three of us stared for a long time at each other. Helen's and Julian's eyes shone, and I felt deeply connected.

The Love of His Sons

I was outside watering the garden when the phone rang. Dropping the hose in a bed of purple verbena, I ran into the kitchen, wiping my hands on my jeans.

"Hullo," I said breathlessly.

"Hi, Mom." Ben's voice said. "You okay?"

"Sure . . . I just ran in from the garden. We leave tomorrow. And I've so much to do."

"Well, I'm calling from New York. I'm visiting Jeff."

"Hey, that's great. I love hearing that you get together."

"So, how's it going?" Ben asked. "We're phoning to see how you're doing before the trip."

I collapsed on a kitchen chair, glad for this respite from my long list of things to do. "Well, I don't know why I'm so nervous. Dad's really excited, but he thinks he has to make a speech. He keeps trying to read old journals and scientific papers."

"That must be hard to watch," Ben said.

"And I know I'll cry. Seeing Dad's friends . . . so many people he's worked with . . ."

Spring 1993

"A lot's going on, Mom. It's great he's being honored by his colleagues at the conference."

"Right. But I feel all jangly. In the Canary Islands we didn't know anyone, really, except Manuel and Maria. And it was all in Spanish. No one knew about Dad's problems. It was a big show. But at the Asilomar conference, we'll know lots of people."

And out poured my fears about Julian not being able to talk, anxiety about awkward moments when I would have to bail him out, sadness over Julian no longer being who he once was.

"I know, Mom, but you'll have friends there," Ben said. "You always get nervous before an event."

"I wish you and Jeff could come. It was great having you in the Canary Islands. You were such a help—running around after Dad, talking to people, keeping conversations going . . ."

"I wish we could be there," Ben said. "Asilomar *is* different. Dad's Alzheimer's will be public. Seven months ago, in the Canary Islands, it was hidden."

Ben was right. My worries about the Tenerife ceremony had to do with presenting an appearance. But the Asilomar award was being given to Julian by the professional organization he'd worked with for years—*because* he had Alzheimer's. It was a public acknowledgment, even though the word "Alzheimer's" would never be mentioned. Suddenly I understood why I was anxious.

"You're a strong woman, Mom. It'll be fine. Want to talk to Jeff?"

"Thanks, Ben. I'll go put Dad on the other phone."

As I walked toward Julian's study holding the portable phone, Jeff's voice came on, so like Ben's: "Mom, how's it going?"

"Jeff, hi! I already told our news to Ben. Ask him to tell you what I said. Wait, I'm getting Dad."

I found Julian sitting at his desk, which was strewn with papers. I handed him the phone. "It's Jeff," I said. "Jeff . . . from New York." He looked at me quizzically and put the phone to his ear upside down. I took it from him and turned it right side up, then went into the bedroom and picked up our second phone. I sank down on the bed, resting and listening.

"Hey, Dad. How're you doing? When are you leaving for your trip?"

Pause. I heard the long silence, determined not to fill it.

"Asilomar," Jeff said. "Aren't you getting an award, Dad? In Asilomar?"

"Yeah . . . uh-huh . . . pretty soon . . . down there . . . we're going to . . . Alzheimer's."

Jeff laughed. "Not Alzheimer's, Dad. Asilomar. You're going to Asilomar. Sounds like Alzheimer's, huh?"

Listening, I smiled. Ironic. Julian can never remember the word "Alzheimer's."

"It's great about your award, Dad." I marveled at how easily Jeff spoke with Julian. He laughed and told him about some weird people he had met on the subway. I could hear the delight in Julian's voice.

"How's that place . . . the big place?"

"You mean New York?"

"No . . . your big place over there."

"Oh, school." And Jeff told about the paper on Mozart he had written for his theory class and how he was getting a scholarship from the music department.

"Wonderful, Jeffy," Julian said.

"Have a great time, Dad. Congratulations on your award. Call me after you get back."

I listened quietly to Jeff talking with Julian, not wanting to interrupt. I appreciated the concern and support I felt from our sons, even though they lived far away and couldn't help in practical ways, as Karen does. Suddenly I remembered the water by now flooding the verbena. I slammed down the phone and ran outside to turn off the hose, thinking whether I should take my black pants *and* my green pants, and which shirt Julian should wear to the banquet.

Julian's Proudest Moment

"You should wear a jacket and tie," Ray Rosen, our old friend and the past president of the International Academy of Sex Researchers, told Julian on the phone before the conference. "After all, you're the guest of honor."

Spring 1993

So Julian and I packed his good sport coat, a nice white shirt, and a striped tie and headed for Asilomar, the state conference center located on a rocky, cypress-studded strip of the northern California coast. We checked into our room in a dark, wooden lodge set on sand dunes and surrounded by tall Monterey pines. We showered, dressed, and met Ray in the dining room as planned.

"Here's our guest of honor," Ray kept introducing Julian to folks assembling for the banquet. Julian had not attended the Academy's meetings for two years, while for years previously he had been a major figure.

Julian had eagerly anticipated this event. Ever since he received the invitation months ago, he had been asking me the date.

"June thirtieth," I kept telling him. "June thirtieth. In two months. Next month. Look in your calendar, it's written there."

Although he had been excited at the letter stating that he was to be honored at the Academy's closing banquet, he had been anxious too. He kept thinking he had to "prepare" for the conference—as he had for so many conferences over his long career. Going to a conference had always meant delivering a lecture, checking last-minute facts, preparing slides, assembling data. He couldn't believe he was going to an international meeting where he didn't have to *do* anything.

"I've got to say something," he kept telling me. "I need to prepare."

"You don't have to *do* anything," I repeated. "You're being honored for your lifetime of work. All you have to do is stand there and say 'Thank you.'"

It took him a long time to realize that he was not attending the scientific sessions, but, rather, the banquet, where he wasn't responsible for talking science.

"Just say 'Thank you,'" I repeated. "No one expects you to give a speech."

But Julian wanted to say something. For months he had fretted over what he should say. Each time I asked what he was thinking about, he couldn't tell me. As the date drew closer, he went to his study to "work on my talk." Day after day he disappeared into the library. One evening he came home for dinner and thrust three pages of handwriting into my hands.

"Here," he said. "I worked on this all day. Maybe you can type it up."

I read through the pages carefully, then read them again. His handwriting looked familiar. It looked okay if you glanced at the pages from a distance. But up close the words didn't make sense. Not one grammatical sentence. Not one comprehensible phrase. No words even that gave me a clue as to what he was trying to say.

Even though I knew he could hardly write anymore, the written gibberish stabbed my heart like a hot poker.

"Darling," I said in bed that night. "I couldn't quite make out the main points of what you wrote. What do you want to say? Tell me and we'll write it together."

Julian snapped off the light and said, "Let's do it in the morning." The next day he said, "I've read over this and it doesn't make sense. I must have been tired. I'll try again today." And off he went to the library, returning home that night and handing me another two pages of writing.

Scanning the paper, this time I made out a few phrases: ". . . it will be a pleasure and joy to come back with and me tu omar see and and attend to the evening of June and its and day. . . . Although I have not in worked in the day most loved and I will be a persual . . . strangely I was finished re this important and pleasure becaus I with . . . strangely I was shong because just at system . . ."

The conference was now only four days away.

"I'll help you," I said. "Let's try something different. Here's the tape recorder. Come sit on the bed and tell me what you want to say to the people at the banquet."

On Sunday morning, for one hour, Julian spoke haltingly, but passionately, about leaving his career. In garbled phrases he described what he felt about science and why he was quitting. He needed his colleagues to know why he had left. He wanted them to know, too, that people with Alzheimer's are still "regular folks."

"I got it," I said.

How clearly he had expressed what was on his mind, not in complete sentences, but I knew what he was trying to say. From talks we had over the years, I understood his intent. I transcribed the tape, typing it into the computer. I eliminated repetitions and clarified awkward phrases, transforming them into appropriate sentences. The vocabulary and sentence structures were mine, but the essence of the message was truly his.

Then I handed Julian the printout to edit, his old, familiar writing routine. This was how he had done all his writing, only his secretary had done the typing. He happily took the pages to the library, returning at night to show me his editing, a word changed here or there, a penciled note in the margin. The corrections made little sense, but the form of his writing routine was comfortably maintained.

Even though we now had a two-page statement, I began to worry. Was this appropriate for the banquet? His words were simple and revealing. They would leave him exposed, vulnerable. This was an international meeting of high-powered scientists, after all.

Julian's colleagues began arriving in California for the conference, and several stopped at our house to visit. I showed the pages to two friends and asked what they thought.

One said with tears in his eyes, "This is a precious gift. Even if I didn't know Julian, I would treasure it. I would feel sorry for anyone who thought it inappropriate." Another said, "The most important thing is for Julian to say whatever he wants. I'll be proud and happy to read it for him."

So, on the evening of the banquet, Julian, looking quite professorial in his white shirt, tweed jacket, and tie, walked into the dining room holding my hand, the two pages neatly folded in my purse. Round tables held wine bottles, candles, and vases of flowers. Julian and I sat with Leonore Teifer, the current president of the International Academy of Sex Researchers, Ray Rosen, the past president, and John Bancroft, a prominent psychiatrist from Edinburgh, the friend who'd volunteered to read Julian's talk.

After dinner Leonore went to the microphone at the front of the room, clapped her hands, and called Julian to stand beside her.

"Now for the main part of the evening," she said, presenting Julian with a bronze plaque. "To Julian Davidson," she read, "in recognition of his distinguished contributions to sexology research."

I sat three tables from the front and could hardly see Julian or Leonore. But I craned my neck and stood from time to time to watch Julian standing handsome and proud, holding the plaque, his curly gray hair, gray beard, and glasses making him look like a wise rabbi.

"Don't go away," Leonore said to Julian. "Several people want to say a few words about you and your work."

Leonore took Julian's elbow, and they stood arm in arm as colleagues and friends went up to the microphone to speak.

Lin Myers, a postdoctoral fellow for two years in Julian's lab, said, "I wanted to work with Julian because I admired the broad scope of his research. He had the 'big look'—the bio-psy-cho-social view which many of us have been talking about at these meetings. Some think this approach is impossible, but I learned from Julian that it *is* possible. I think this is the most important of his many contributions."

She went on to say, "There are some Julian stories you *can* tell and some you *can't* tell." Laughter burst from the audience. Then she told one "Julian story" involving going to the anatomy lab down the hall to take some measurements. The lab technician handed them a dissected groin, and they carefully measured various sections of the cadaver's penis.

"It was fun working in Julian's lab," she said above the laughter. "Research is fun. Sex is fun. And sex research is really fun. I learned this from Julian very well. I also learned," she said, her voice taking on a more sober tone, "that we need to respect our human, and nonhuman, subjects. And respect ourselves as well. Most important," she said, "we need to honor each other . . . while we're here."

Loud applause accompanied her as she sat down. I wiped a tear from my eye and saw others wadding up tissues as well.

Leonore took the mike. "I have a special bond with Julian,"

she said as the next speaker approached, "unlike anyone else in this room. I've known Julian since 1964, when we met accidentally at the founding convention of the Peace and Freedom Party." Over the laughter I shouted "Yay, Peace 'n' Freedom!" remembering how I had been the first registrar of voters for that fledgling group in our county. "Yay, Peace 'n' Freedom!" I yelled, feeling giddy from chardonnay and the occasion.

"So many wonderful stories about Julian come to mind," said Ray Rosen, in his crisp South African accent, "but I would like to tell two tonight from the sabbatical year I spent in Julian's lab in 1989, a privilege and a pleasure. We've talked many times during this meeting of the tremendous impact of Julian's work on the field, so I would like to share some anecdotes about his character."

And Ray described how his family had been taken aback by West Coast life after moving from New Jersey. One example was the invitation by Stanford president Donald Kennedy to attend a "jazz Shabbat," sent to all the Jewish faculty. "Julian and my family went together," Ray said.

"Both of us were brought up in traditional Jewish families, and we were curious. In the middle of this strange Sabbath service, all set to jazz, Julian turned to me and asked, 'What exactly is going on here?' Underneath Julian's reputation as a far-out sex researcher, he is really quite a conservative chappie. It was the best Sabbath service either of us ever attended.

"A more touching and serious memory from that year," Ray continued, "was the big Loma Prieta earthquake—October 17, 1989. My family and I had just arrived a few days before. Two things stand out: Julian's incredible efforts to keep his research projects going despite the damage and shutdown of the wonderful old Anatomy Building, which housed his lab. And the incredible love, generosity, and hospitality Julian and Ann extended after the quake. The lights were out, the water was off, and aftershocks shook every few minutes. My wife, two small sons, and I ran to their house, scared and shaken. Julian and Ann immediately said, 'Stay with us, don't worry, we'll open some cans, light candles, and eat dinner together.' Julian's been a wonderful colleague and a wonderful friend. I hope we'll have many years together!"

Next, Barry Komisaruk took the mike and spoke about the evolution of Julian's career. "There's a facet of Julian Davidson's career that you sex researchers here might not be aware of," he said. "Julian is also one of the most gifted neuroendocrinologists in the field. In the 1950s and 1960s, Julian contributed some brilliant studies on the mechanisms by which the brain controls the pituitary gland, gonads, and adrenals. He was one of the main contributors to a burgeoning new field. Then he became involved in how the brain controls behavior, first in animal studies and later in studies of human sexual behavior.

"Julian was a great role model," Barry said, "because I saw it was possible to study human sexual behavior in the tradition of medical physiology and neuroendocrinology. You should all be aware that Julian is one of the most respected neuroendocrinologists, apart from his later great contributions to human sexuality."

Richard Green, a noted psychiatrist and sex researcher who has known Julian for thirty years, affirmed Barry's comments. "Very few people, if any, have made the transition from laboratory physiology to human sexuality," he said. "Julian's transition is remarkable."

"This is the part of the meeting I've looked forward to most," he added, giving Julian a hug before handing the microphone to John Bancroft, host of next year's conference.

"I'm going to say a few words from me and then I'm going to say a few words from Julian," John said in his precise British accent, motioning for Julian to come stand beside him.

"You've all heard about Julian's very unusual, if not unique, contributions to our science. One of the things I'm particularly proud about in my career is when Julian decided to come to my lab in Edinburgh." Then he told, in a perfectly dry academic tone, how he and Julian had "stuck suppositories of dihydrotestosterone . . . up our bums." Howls of laughter drowned out whatever else he said about that.

Pausing for the laughter to quiet, he said solemnly, "Julian is keen to get a message across. This is a very emotional occasion. For that reason I think he felt it might be a bit difficult for him, so he asked me to do it. These are Julian's words."

In a slow, clear voice, his face sober, controlling his own emotions, John read:

First of all, I want to thank Leonore for her kind remarks and thank the Academy for this honor. I am happy to be here to see many old friends.

As most of you know, I am no longer working in the field. I'll officially retire from Stanford next month. I would like to take this opportunity to make a few comments about what I've been learning since I stopped working at the old science game.

I enjoyed my work for thirty years. It was fun, enjoyable, and, I hope, useful too. I've made many good friends. But some years ago, my work began to be increasingly difficult. I began to think slowly and wasn't as quick at remembering.

At first, I noticed these changes, but I didn't understand why the work wasn't going well. Eventually the doctors diagnosed me as having memory problems, which explained what I had for years been observing. As I gradually saw that the work wasn't as good as it had been, I didn't want to continue. Slowly I understood that I needed to stop my old work and begin a new life . . . which isn't easy.

Although I looked forward to doing other things, I felt sorry about losing my career. I felt sad to leave the work which has been a major part of my life. At the same time, I felt excited about changing my life. I also had to learn to accept what the doctors told me.

Those of you who have talked with me may notice my problems. One example is talking. I can speak, but not well, and not in groups. People talk too fast. Another problem is that everything feels slow and complicated. Some things are impossible and not worth trying.

So I face the challenge of learning to be a new and different kind of person. I must accept there are many things I can't do. Even so, I have a pretty full life, only with no science in it. Something unimaginable a few years ago. But it's amazing what you can adjust to. I want you to know that although some parts of my brain don't work, I'm the same guy. I still enjoy a rewarding life.

So, yes, I'm retired. And I accept the challenge of adjusting to these changes. Now that I'm out, I do different things: I volunteer at the Food Closet, giving food to homeless people. I work in an organic vegetable garden on a nearby farm. I'm an active member of Parents and Friends of Lesbians and Gays. I sing in a Yiddish chorus, go to concerts, and swim, run, bike ride, and hike. Hard to imagine myself in a life without science, but there you are. . . ."

A lump rose in my throat. I sat quietly in my seat staring at the flickering candle on the center of the table. Briefly I stood up to catch a glimpse of John and Julian. Julian stood next to John, holding his plaque to his chest, a solemn expression on his face. The room was silent. All the extraneous chatter and side remarks had stopped. John's voice quivered slightly but remained controlled and filled with respect. I hoped Julian felt all right.

John's soft voice continued reading.

My brain ain't what it used to be. I also have arthritis in my big toes. But I want you to know that, in between, everything works just fine!

Laughter exploded from the audience. People jumped to their feet and applauded. The entire room stood and clapped. The applause went on and on, this last remark relieving the hushed tension. The applause faded as John concluded.

Once again, it's great to be here. And thank you for welcoming and honoring me at this banquet.

As soon as John finished, the audience again leapt to their feet. They shouted and whooped. They clapped and clapped. I couldn't see Julian. I also stood and applauded, letting the applause wash over me as I hoped he was letting it wash over him—this well-deserved recognition from his colleagues. How much this must mean to him.

Ironically, the celebration fell on the very evening before his official retirement from Stanford, this day he had been inching toward with such hope and dread. The applause continued. I could see people bringing out tissues. Then the music began. The band pounded out the beat, and couples moved onto the dance floor.

I pushed through the crowd toward Julian at the front of the room, where a group clustered around him admiring the bronze inscription. I went to him, hugged and kissed him. We lay the plaque on the table and began to dance. Finding the beat, we lost ourselves to the rhythm. Drunk with wine and pleasure, we swayed and stomped and twirled. The evening went by in a whirl of dancing, talking, hugging, laughing.

People came up to me, many with tears in their eyes, some I recognized and some I didn't know. They told me about Julian, experiences they had shared, aspects of his work.

"Julian's work was at the cutting edge," one said. "He asked the right questions at the right time. He was creative in designing experiments to answer those questions."

Another told me, his eyes moist with tears, "Julian was a great teacher . . . my role model."

Another said he was such a clear writer. He could assimilate many disparate facts and make sense of them. His writing covered a big field. He straddled and integrated different disciplines.

A blond woman I didn't know asked me how Julian is, what he does all day and how I cope. Her voice quivered. Her eighty-eight-year-old father had Alzheimer's, she told me, and she doesn't know how to be with him. He used to be smart, she said, but now they have only simple conversations.

"And he's my father, not my husband." She looked at me as if I might have some answers.

"Well," I said, as we walked outside to escape the loud music, "I try to stay present in each moment. If I look back and think of the man that he was, the man I have lost, it's too sad. I'm overwhelmed with loss and grief. If I look ahead to what may come in the future, it's too frightening to imagine."

I looked up at the myriad of stars in the dark night sky. "But if I stay present, moment by moment, it isn't so bad. Each day has its blessings and pleasures. I try to reach for what's healthy in Julian. I reach for what's normal and relate to that part, however small it may be. I try to love and protect him. He deserves love, care, fun, and understanding. He can't help the fact that he's leaving.

"I also cry and I scream sometimes too. Some days are very hard," I added. She stared at my face as I spoke.

Back on the dance floor, Julian took off his jacket and loos-ened his tie. He danced with abandon, arms and legs flopping loosely, in his old sixties, carefree style. Then he took off his tie and rolled up his sleeves.

The guest of honor danced and danced—with me, with Leonore, with Lin Myers, and with the blond woman I didn't know.

As midnight approached and the band declared its final song, I reached out my hand to John Bancroft and his wife, who were dancing near us. The four of us formed a small circle and pranced around. Then we opened the circle to bring in Ray Rosen, then Lin and Barry, and our circle grew. Around and around we danced in a kind of ill-defined Jewish hora to a rock beat.

Somehow everyone on the dance floor spontaneously joined hands. Forming a long line, we snaked our way in a labyrinth under each other's upheld arms, kicking and skipping and parad-ing around until suddenly we opened into a huge circle, moving, faster and faster, to the escalating crescendo. A wide grin stretched across Julian's glowing face.

Then the band stopped. Midnight, June 30. Suddenly it was July 1, the first day of Julian's retirement. Waitresses began clear-ing the tables and the crowd drifted off. Cradling the plaque, Julian and I walked arm in arm across the white sand dunes to our room, hot from the exuberance of dance and the tributes of friends. Dropping our clothes on the floor beside the bed, we held each other close in the darkness, before falling on the sheets, cling-ing to each other, rolling and tumbling together in love and, soon after, into the long, cool sleep.

A Journey of Love

It's nearly three years since the Asilomar banquet, over five since our journey began.

This morning Julian sat on our bedroom floor, weeping, sur-rounded by a pile of socks. He put on brown ones. Then he pulled them off and put on gray ones. Then he pulled them off, held up a black one, and started to cry. Deciding which to wear was just too much.

Usually I get up before Julian and lay out his clothes. We've evolved a morning routine which works—for now. I shower first while he makes the bed, a task he can still do. The sheets aren't tucked in and blankets form lumps, but he manages to pull the spread over the pillows.

Then I call him into the shower as I step out. This way the water temperature is already set and I can reach in to hand him the soap and pour shampoo on his hair while I'm still wet.

While he showers, I lay his underwear and socks on the bathroom counter, squeeze Crest on his toothbrush, and get out his electric shaver, which I just bought, because using a regular razor and shaving cream, as he's always done, is now impossible. Then I leap into my underwear and lie on the carpet in sunlight which streams in through our bedroom window, trying to do my back exercises and a few yoga postures before he appears.

Sometimes he comes in and steps on my outstretched arm or bumps into my leg. Sometimes he comes naked into the room, struggling to put his foot into his undershirt instead of underpants, looking at me with a puzzled expression. Often I must leave my "dog pose" and hand him his underpants or stop him from brushing his hair with the toothbrush.

Always he is talking.

"We've got to get the ma-vee up to the laboree. The laby . . . the lobby . . . there's a nice man up there on the animal, you know. I want to go to the labee and if it doesn't work . . . in the faber of the meevay. We could . . . you understand?"

"We could," I might answer. Or, "That's interesting," or "No, I didn't know that," or "Um-hum."

More and more we perform our "dance of conversation." He speaks and I comment, nod and answer him, though no logical information is exchanged. If I am calm, peaceful, and sound pleasant, Julian is cheerful and satisfied. But it's a demanding role.

"The mavee is in the laboree and we can go after yesterday in the morning."

"Yes, that's true," I might say, but sometimes I am agreeing to something that later doesn't happen and then he questions me for hours, only there's no hope of ever sorting it out.

Alzheimer's, A Love Story

My statements to him now consist of constantly orienting him to time, space, and task. "Put on your sock," or "Let's fix breakfast," or "We're going to visit my father." Each phrase is repeated over and over. If I ask him to hand me a cup, he may take off his shoe. If I tell him to come to the kitchen, he goes to the closet.

Julian doesn't speak pure gibberish, like the man in the Alzheimer's Couples' Group who so frightened me four years ago, the man who said only, "dibika, dibika." But Julian's sentences rarely make sense and increasingly he invents words. "We need the ved . . . after the wating," he says.

By the time Julian and I reach the kitchen, I'm usually tense. But we muddle forward. I listen to news on the radio as I lay out cereal and juice. Sometimes he "helps," if I hand him the bowls and point to the table. But, often as not, he forgets midway between cupboard and table what he is doing, and the bowls end up on the telephone answering machine or in the family room on the TV.

When I finally get him to day care, where he now goes twice a week, I am exhausted. He has trouble opening and closing the car door. I have to put on his seat belt for him. He talks continuously all the way to the day care center which, to my great surprise and relief, he enjoys. He goes cheerfully and is happy, if I pick him up by three.

I'm still not used to seeing him with white-haired folks in wheelchairs and walkers. Some women sit in rocking chairs cradling baby dolls. Some elderly men slump in wheelchairs with bibs tied under their chins to catch their drooling. Other "participants," as they are called, wander about or talk to themselves or are silent. But slowly I see them as real individuals; I chat with them and smile. Each was once a competent adult with a rich past, as is Julian. They all deserve affection and respect.

The day care staff, bless them, greet Julian warmly each morning; create music, art, and exercise programs; and give him a hug when he leaves.

"Julian is wonderful," they tell me. "He's so sweet and gentle and friendly."

Spring 1993

They say he enjoys his day and enthusiastically plays ball, sings, and takes part in "Current Events." Most of all, he praises the desserts.

"You just go there and they give you sweets and no money," Julian says often about the center.

"You're lucky to have him, he's such a nice man," the staff says. And so, in many ways, I am. He's rarely hostile, depressed, belligerent, angry, paranoid, or resistant, as are many others. Not now, anyway.

Each Alzheimer's patient has a unique character. Some may have personality changes. For others, their basic nature remains. Is this due to biochemical whimsy? Are different parts of the brain affected? Does a person's Alzheimer's behavior represent their essential self? Does it reflect how they feel and are handled? I have asked these questions many times and received no clear answers.

For the most part, thankfully, Julian is content, as long as I remain pleasant and organize the day so that he is occupied. After day care, he likes coming with me to do our errands; he enjoys pushing the market basket and carrying the grocery bags to the car. Later we walk in the hills behind Stanford or along the marshes by the bay.

I am no longer shocked by his peculiar language and odd acts. He's forgotten how to turn off lights and flush the toilet. He's forgotten that his sweater goes under his parka, and he wears his pajama top over his shirt. I just notice all this and let it go. Over breakfast in a restaurant yesterday, he poured salt on the butter which came with his pancakes and then slid the whole yellow ball in his mouth with a knife. In a Chinese restaurant last week, he managed to pierce and eat all his Szechuan vegetables with one chopstick, no easy feat.

Recently I realized that our life now matches the lives I had glimpsed in the couples' group after Julian's diagnosis, over five years ago. Julian goes to day care; his language barely makes sense; I can't leave him alone: all this I had watched before with awe and admiration. We have come to exactly the place I so feared.

I can't say life is good, but it isn't as unbearable as it seemed then. Our life is "do-able" and still has daily pleasures. The brave words I uttered that long-ago day in the psychiatrist's office shine before me and hold me to their promise. "Not fear and anger," I had told the doctor. "I want to go down with love."

It's not easy. As I told the blond woman at Asilomar, some days I want to scream "Shut up" when Julian rambles on about the "ved" and the "meevay," when he follows me about the house talking and I can't understand. I feel I'll go crazy if he says "laboree" one more time. Some days I despair over our shrunken little life, and often I can't wait to drop him at day care or for a friend to take him off my hands. Will I get through this? What will be left of me when it is done?

But mostly I feel a tenderness for Julian beyond words. In bed he still rubs my back. We still walk hand in hand in purple twilight shadows by the bay. His face lights up when he sees chocolate. Last week he whistled as we cross-country skied across glistening snow. He managed to ski intermediate trails, even though at night, returning from the bathroom, he not only went into our friends' bedroom, but he actually climbed into their bed. Yesterday he looked long into my eyes and told me he loved me.

Julian, now supervised by two compassionate friends, still goes to the Food Closet. He hums along weekly with the Yiddish Chorus; words no longer matter. Another friend brings a video and fudge cake on Thursday nights and stays with Julian while I run the gay support group meetings. Karen invites her dad for occasional weekends, managing to care for him as well as Antar, Celina, and our new grandbaby. Jeff speaks regularly to us from New York, and Ben visits as often as he can, accompanying Julian to the men's room in restaurants and adding his upbeat presence to outings. Every Monday we dance in Beiçola's samba class, where Julian bounces about like an old hippie to the throbbing beat.

I remembered, when Julian was diagnosed, my panic that everyone would abandon us and that I'd be alone with a crazy man. Instead, the open hearts of our children and friends form strands in the net of support which holds us.

Spring 1993

A winsome, adorable side of Julian emerges as his intellect dwindles. If I truly let go of needing anything from him, an appealing beauty shines forth. He is as transparent and lovable as a two-year-old, irrepressibly funny, living with fewer and fewer inhibitions. The other day, wearing earphones and listening to Vivaldi, he waved his arms wildly about, "conducting" the entire *Four Seasons*. Watching him immersed in pleasure brought tears to my eyes and to Ben's.

Our life pushes on, shrinking and shrinking . . . yet with happy moments despite the dreadful losses. Though some days I crumple with fatigue and doubt, mostly I am confident that I can manage whatever comes, even the dreaded nursing-home decision which lies ahead. I avoid thinking about the day when Julian may no longer know me. I am wedded to the challenge of living with him in a gentle way until our life together comes to whatever its end. I travel in full light, knowing the intense joys and sorrowful griefs of this Alzheimer's journey. There is no way for me to do it, but with love.